3 Week Slim Down Challenge

Pamela Taylor

DEDICATION

This book is dedicated to the amazing people, who read my blog and shared the menus that were organized to help me lose weight after my 3rd child. Seeing that a simple list of easy menu items and shopping list was helping people, has been inspiring me for years to create more menus and support systems. This book is dedicated to your continuous journey for better health, and your individual story of success.

CONTENTS

ACKNOWLEDGMENTS

Thank you for my family that puts up with my dreams and desires to serve others more every year. I know that they have given up time to allow me the freedom to fail and succeed.

I want to also thank my friend and biggest health encourager, Stacey Howell. Her health journey is ever evolving and the level of educating herself to overcome anything has given me so much insight into my own journey as well as ideas to add to my blog & support community.

NOTICE

This book is intended as a reference document only, not as a medical manual. The information given here is designed to help you make shopping and planning for a healthy lifestyle quicker and easier. It is not intended as a substitute for any treatment that may have been prescribed by your doctor. If you suspect that you have a medical problem, I urge you to speak with a medical professional to get help with your specific circumstance.

CHAPTER 1: GETTING STARTED

I hope you're excited as I am that you've chosen to start this 3-week slim down challenge!

You'll be surprised and encouraged at how quickly you can change your health when you focus on the right things, have a simple strategy, and a plan to get there. This book is not about pills, fads, trends or any crazy restrictive diet. It has simple example shopping lists and menus so that you can easily and quickly start your journey today!

This book is not full of difficult to understand medical advice and/or new theories that take you several chapters to comprehend. It is about your personal journey and your daily challenges to improve your health and fitness.

Sometimes people say, "I can do anything for 3 weeks", or "I can do anything for one week". But I'd love for you to think that you can do anything for just one day. Take this challenge one day at a time. Every day wake up as if it's a new day and you can make new decisions. This way you don't fall into the trap of making one mistake one day and deciding to start all over with the challenge. Don't be quick to decide it's not working for you. One part of the challenge is every day do something for your health, both mentally and physically. We'll talk more about how the two are intertwined in the next chapter.

Improving your health has more to do with how you think and the food you eat than how much time you spend at the gym. Unfortunately, our society pushes weight loss programs that are in the supplement industry, exercise videos, and gyms that are making billions.

The sad truth is, most gyms make a lot of money off of people that don't show up. In addition, the supplement industry is full of bad information. There is probably some minimal truth to their claims and statements, but if you read the risks and disclosures, it's downright terrifying a lot of supplements. Therefore, when someone ask me what supplements or appetite suppressants I recommend, my answer typically is water. Staying hydrated and drinking water is the number one simple healthy habit you can do. No matter how much money, technology, or resources you have, water is the easiest habit that will improve your experience.

Again, I'm really excited you decided to take the 3-week slim down challenge. It's all about your health, help, and support. It is not a lot of fluff, so we'll get right to it.

Before we start, I would love to connect with you and learn more about you through the challenge questions and our community. I'm very open with my email, and I love to connect, serve, and support you as much as I can.

Let's be friends!

EMAIL:

FACEBOOK: https://www.facebook.com/removemyweight

FB support Group:
https://www.facebook.com/groups/myweightlosscommunity

INSTAGRAM: https://www.instagram.com/removemyweight

TWITTER: https://www.twitter.com/removemyweight

PINTEREST: https://www.pinterest.com/removemyweight

BLOG: https://www.removemyweight.com/blog

Personal Thoughts
(Questions, that you hope are answered over the next 3-weeks.)

____

____

____

____

____

____

____

List the reasons why you are ready to lose weight, now.

1.____

2.____

3.____

4.____

5.____

6.____

CHAPTER 2: HOW TO USE THIS BOOK

Simplicity is key

This book is made to be simple. There are plenty of people out there that are making dieting and overall health complicated. This book is not going to take you a week to read through and/or 30 minutes to an hour for any given recipe or shopping list. This is meant to make weight loss and being healthy as simple as possible.

Less than 5 minutes (of prep) a day simple.

We'll let all those other books that are 300+ pages long and go into medical theory and research take care of your desire to go into more depth on individual things.

Instead, I'll give you the tools, a guide, and some simple plans to really focus on your journey. What you learn about yourself and what you learn about food is all a benefit to making significant changes.

There are literally millions of blog posts and books on health and nutrition and all the individual characteristics of every food. If you go online and google the word "Apple" you will find hundreds of thousands of links directly related to telling you how good or bad it is for your overall health. We're not going to mess with any of that information because there are people far more educated than me to give you specifics and micro-nutrition facts on all foods and/or health conditions. Therefore, the menus and foods listed in this book are generalized and a good reference for most. Try to focus on maximizing your healthy choices, changes in your food, and healthy habits. That is where a lot of poor health can be turned around.

Example menus

We have more than 3 weeks of example menus (chapter 10) and a huge list of foods that are exchangeable (chapter 9). A shopping list to take to the grocery store with you, so you can easily get great healthy foods for your body. These menus are to serve as an example and reference of what I've used in my own journey and others have shown interest in by being shared over 50,000 times on Pinterest and other sources. There are hundreds of other menus by calorie count on my website.

https://www.removemyweight.com

You're welcome to check it out and download other free menus or join as a member and get 100s of more menus within seconds.

In fact, if you write an honest review of this book and/or send me proof of purchase, such as a picture of you holding the book or a receipt, I will give you free access on my website to the hundreds of menus in our preferred area. In addition, you can do this 3-Week Slim Down Challenge online, by email and with our support group.

In our community we have people starting this challenge almost every day. There is a lot of questions answered. Feel free to join us at
https://www.facebook.com/groups/myweightlosscommunity/

This book is truly dedicated to you and your success. Since every journey is so personal, and everyone is starting at a different point you'll get a few references of the best diet to start, but for the most part you must pay attention to your body and make good decisions from there.

The menus provided in the back of this book are approximately 1200 calories per day. This is a good amount for many people to lose weight at a steady pace (which is typically understood at half a pound to two pounds a week).

Many men may need to stay ~1500 calories per day or above and women that are more than 40 pounds overweight. This can be achieved by simply doubling the meat quantity, on any of the example menus provided.

With that being said, if you know how many calories you typically eat, per day, on a regular basis, subtract around 500 calories from that amount you should be able to lose 1 pound a week. If you are unsure of how many calories to eat per day to lose weight, you can use the Calorie Counter on the website to get an estimate.

https://www.removemyweight.com/calorie-calculator.html

Journal pages

The journal pages are designed for you to write down what food you're eating so that you can count calories and keep yourself accountable.

The journal pages are broken up into six categories.
1) Goals & Healthy Habits
2) Food Journal
3) Fitness and Water
4) Notes
5) Improvement Ideas
6) Gratitude Journal

Category 1 - Your To-Do List Goals and Healthy Habits.

This is to be filled out at the beginning of every day if possible. It's good to write down some of the goals you have for the day. These can be personal, spiritual, family or health-related goals. If you write down your goals, you're far more likely to get them done. It's a good step at the beginning of every day to document what you want from your day. The next part of the section is healthy habits. In most societies we do not get enough vitamins from our food even if we're doing our best, so it's recommended to take a simple multivitamin or if you know certain vitamins that you need to stay healthy.

Getting more than seven hours of sleep is a good check. Sometimes it will help you look back on the days that you got less sleep. When you make poor food decisions or are low on energy, it's easy to not make the smartest health choices. When we exercise, if we didn't get proper sleep, we're not getting the biggest benefit out of it, so it's always good to track.

It's also good to have some quiet time and depending on your personal faith that maybe prayer, meditation, maybe just taking a bath, or spending a little more time in the shower. Taking some time every day even if it's one, five, or thirty minutes is a good practice to really focus on improving yourself and mental clarity. This quiet time for reflection and relaxation is really a great habit.

Category 2 - Your Food Journal.

The second portion of the journal is your food journal. This is where we keep a simple list and not make it overcomplicated of what foods you eat and the approximate calories. Do not over concern yourself with being exact on calories whether it's 90 calories or 110 it's probably not going to make much of a difference. On the other hand, if you had a candy bar, be honest.

You can use the approximate calories on the example menus and/or alternate options in chapter 9. You will make different choices if you have to physically write it down and look at it later. When you look at what you eat compared to how you feel and how much sleep you got, you may notice a pattern. Consistency will help educate you on your own health decisions and choices.

If you cheat on this challenge, it is not meant to make you feel bad or guilty. It's just for you to be able to document and review your healthy choices and unhealthy choices. Snacks are optional but in general, if you feel like a snack, have one between breakfast and lunch or between lunch and dinner. Be very careful about snacking too much after 8 PM. It typically isn't necessary, and you'll realize you're emotional eating rather than eating for nutritional needs.

Category 3 - Your Fitness and Water habits.

The next section is your fitness and water intake. There is space to mark down how many minutes that you spent on your overall exercise. This could be weight training or cardio. You do not have to exercise to lose weight. With that being said, fitness has far more benefits than just weight-loss and it will aid in making your body stronger and healthier. The last time I met with my doctor she recommended 30 minutes of exercise 3 to 5 times a week and 15+ minutes of weight training type exercises at least twice a week. The biggest advantage of fitness and health is making it into a daily habit. Being honest with yourself if you think you don't have time. Everybody has one minute to do either jumping jacks or a few push-ups. Even one minute a day is better than nothing.

Within this section is water intake. There're are eight spots for 8 cups of water, and if you drink more than that you'll see you more health benefits. Water helps your body filter toxins as your body burns fat, and it has so many other benefits. One of the biggest is that it will help you feel full. Many people mistake being thirsty for being hungry. Sometimes if you are starting to feel a little hungry, before you reach for food, drink a cup of water. You may find that it helps your cravings more than the food would have.

Category 4 - Your Thoughts and Feelings.

The next section is for you to write notes on your day. Try to be honest but try to be positive. A lot of times on a health journey we tend to feel critical and guilty, instead of positive. If you stopped eating after 8 PM, make sure you give yourself credit for that. If you walked past the popcorn counter at the movies, that is a huge celebration, especially if that was a negative habit. If you happen to get popcorn but only had a small instead of a large, chalk that up to a win. We are all still starting from a different place and you need to celebrate every small win and change that you see in your day. This is also where you can reflect on the daily challenges, and any tips that you want to remember.

Category 5 - Your Improvement Opportunities.

The next section is improvement ideas. Rather than focus on what you may have done wrong, mistakes or the backpedals that happened throughout the day. Focus on areas you can improve. If you work from home sometimes the fridge can be a concern and you need to give some rules for yourself. One easy rule is to only eat in the kitchen and not next to your computer. This is good advice whether you work from home or in an office. The goal is to change your habits to be consistent with your health goals rather than just give yourself a lot of rules and restrictions.

Category 6 – Your Gratitude List.

The next section is gratitude. It is very important to be grateful for the things in your life. A positive attitude can do wonders for your overall health. For example, every day I am grateful that my kids wake up healthy, I'm grateful that I have two arms, two legs, and I can go to the gym no matter what excuses I can come up with. We all have people in our life that have significant restrictions. There are things that they can't do that we can, even in our current circumstance. It's important to be grateful for that. Be appreciative of the little things like a phone call from a friend. Time is a gift that's always fleeting. This can be part of your quiet time, or meditation practice and/or prayer time. As you're developing better health habits, it's good to keep your mind positive and remember how many good things you have in life, because the world is more than happy to show us the negative.

Personal Thoughts

(Inspiration, that you hope will keep you motivated for 3-weeks.)

____

____

____

____

____

____

How will you feel after 3-weeks?

(List those feelings, and start feeling them now.)

____

____

____

____

____

____

____

CHAPTER 3: DON'T LISTEN TO ME

Why listen to me, I'm not a "health coach" …

I want to tell you a story about a time I was talking to a friend. I stated something to the fact of "I hate cooking'. She replies, "Yeah, my family eats a lot of fast food too".

I was a little shocked at her response because she had completely misunderstood what I said. I didn't say I *don't* cook. In fact, I cook all the time, but I don't "*enjoy*" cooking.

Some people love the process of creating something beautiful and yummy for their family. Some people relish in the art of mixing multiple ingredients to get the flavor just right. Maybe they love the hours of chopping, and using every dish in the kitchen, for that perfect dinner dish.

I'm on the other side of that, I like eating healthy foods and providing a healthy meal for my family. But nothing frustrates me more than recipes that are 20 ingredients long (10 being spices) and take several hours to prepare.

The average diet cookbook is at least 10-15 ingredients for every "simple dish". My idea of a simple dish is just a few ingredients.

It always pains me, that so many weight-loss programs require hours and hours of effort every day to get any results. I designed the menus in this book to be so easy that you spend only 30 minutes at the store every week and have healthy foods that help you stay full. Your pre-calorie counted, nutritious menu plan examples are designed so that you can lose weight without too much extra work. Nothing on the ingredients list take me more than five minutes to prepare, and you can use whatever seasonings you like as long as it's not a stick of butter.

Seasoning mixes provide plenty of variation and can eliminates hundreds of dollars' worth of spices necessary for those fancy homemade rubs. Mesquite barbecue, rotisserie chicken, salt, pepper, and steak seasoning will do amazing things to the flavor of your dishes.

A word of warning, if you love to spend hours and hours in the kitchen daily preparing wonderful meals for your family and/or yourself, these plans will probably not fit your interest. On the other hand, if you're like most people, time-starved and just really want a simple plan that's easily adjusted for an individual or a family and fits your nutritional needs, these menu plans might be perfect for you.

Picture This….

A woman with new 8-week baby in her arms, 4 hours of sleep, a 1-year old dumping out the toy bin, a 3-year old asking where her favorite doll is, all while she is trying to get ready for work. If you can picture this, you probably feel the same overwhelming exhaustion that she did.

This was my story, and trust me, finding time for the gym was not at the top of my priority list. I was lucky if I got out of the house without the kids more than an hour a week.

Maybe you can relate to the exhaustion of taking care of everything and everyone more than yourself. I gained 50 pounds with each child and it wasn't as easy losing weight in my 30s, as it was in my 20s. I was in the perfect mindset for all those late-night infomercials, with their weight loss programs. The problem is, that almost all of them want you to workout 30 minutes or more a day or buy their food "system". I didn't feel like I had the time, nor did I feel like I could justify the expense of the packaged food programs.

Oh, to top things off, I'd had back surgery in my late 20s and therefore my workout choices were limited. In addition to that, every side of my family health history has type 2 diabetes, therefore I'm not pre-dispositioned to be thin if you know what I mean.

I was determined to not use my kids, busy life, or my family history as an excuse for my health or weight. I needed an easy, effective, and real plan. So, I researched all the information I could on nutrition and weight loss.

The crazy thing is, it's not that complicated: 80% of weight loss success is as simple as the foods we eat. My question is this: Why do most all weight loss plans talk more about exercise than foods when **your shopping list is the key to your weight loss?**

I get it, everyone wants a bikini body, but most of us would be happy if our pants fit. You know, that one pair in the back of your closet that someday, you will fit into again. The fact is, first you need to get a handle on your foods. Knowing what to eat and having a plan is the fastest, easiest, and 'least sweaty' way to health.

I created this book and all of the online resources to help with simple menus that truly remove all excuses because it is not that hard to follow.

CHAPTER 4: PRE- SURVEY

Date _________________________________

Who shops for food at your home?

____

Who prepares it? _____________________________

What do you drink during the day?

____

What kind of meat do you usually buy?

___ beef, steak, pork chops   ___ chicken, turkey, fish

If you don't eat meat, what types of protein do you buy?

____

What type of meal or meals do you prepare most often?

___ fry   ___ bake   ___ broil   ___ slow cook   ___ grill

How many times a day do you eat?

____

What do you usually eat?

____

How many times do you **eat out** during the week?

____

What restaurant do you go to most often?

____

List any vitamins or dietary supplements you take. How
many of each do you take? How often?

____

If you eat any special foods for health or personal reasons,
list what kind and how much

____

List any medication you take (prescription or over the
counter). How many of each do you take? How often?

____

Do you feel well rested and excited for the day? If not how
often do you feel that way?

____

How healthy do you feel (on a scale of 1 to 10, 1 = terrible)?

____

Do you feel optimistic about the next month? If so why?

____

Pre-Challenge Measurements

Before you start measuring, remember to:

- Use a non-stretchable tape
- Make sure the tape measure is level around your body and parallel to the floor
- Keep the tape close to your skin without depressing it.

Measurements:

- o **Bust/ Upper Chest:** Measure all the way around your bust and back on the line of your nipples.
- o **Chest:** Measure directly under your breasts, as high up as possible.
- o **Waist:** Measure at its narrowest point width-wise, usually just above the navel.
- o **Hips:** Measure around the widest part of the hipbones.
- o **Upper arm:** Measure above your elbows – around fullest part.
- o **Thighs:** Measure around fullest part of upper leg while standing
- O **Calves:** Measure around fullest part.

Weigh-In

Measurement	Start
Body Fat %	
Upper Chest	
Chest	
Waist	
Stomach	
Hips	
Left Upper Arm	
Right Upper Arm	
Right Thigh	
Left Thigh	
Right Calf	
Left Calf	

Survey: Your Typical Servings in a Week

Dairy

____ glass(es) (8 ounces) of whole milk

____ glass(es) of 2% milk or 1% or skim milk

____ 1 ounce slice(s) of cheese

____ serving(s) of yogurt or cottage cheese

Vegetables

____ scoop-sized helping(s) of vegetables

____ small vegetable salad(s)

____ medium-sized potato(es)

Fruits

____ piece(s) of fruit (an apple, orange, banana, slice of melon, etc.)

____ 1/2 cup(s) cooked or canned fruit

Meat

____ small piece(s) of meat, fish, or poultry (about the size of a deck of cards)

____ 2 eggs

____ 1 cup(s) cooked dried beans or peas

____ 4 tablespoons peanut butter

_____ This page totals

Survey: Your Typical Servings in a Week

Grains

_____ slice(s) of bread or tortilla(s)

_____ small roll(s), biscuit(s), or muffin(s)

_____ 1/2 bun(s), English muffin(s), or bagel(s)

_____ cooked cereal, rice, or pasta

_____ small bowl(s) of cold cereal

Sweets and Fats

_____ 10 chips or french fries

_____ candy bar(s) or 3 small cookies

_____ slice(s) of pie or cake

_____ sweet roll(s) or donut(s)

_____ 1/2 cup(s) of ice cream

_____ rounded teaspoon(s) of margarine or butter

_____ tablespoon(s) of salad dressing

_____ Pizza, spaghetti, lasagna, or Mac and Cheese

Drinks

_____ 12-ounce soda drinks

_____ glass(es) of Kool-Aid or fruit punch

_____ energy drinks

_____ 12-ounce beer(s)

_____ 4 ounces of wine (small glass)

_____ shot(s) of liquor (1.5 oz.)

_____ This page totals

CHAPTER 5: DAY 0 - SHOPPING

Welcome to the 3 Week Slim Down!! I'm absolutely THRILLED you are reading this.

It's important to get a few things done before you start, whether you are starting tomorrow, or in a few days from now. Start when you want, just don't stop until the 3 weeks are up.

3 STEP SET-UP:

STEP 1: **Pick your Menu Plan for the next 7 Days.**

There are 5 weeks of example menus with shopping lists in Chapter 10. In a couple of pages, there is a simple starter menu that works great to help ease into this challenge. Then, go Shopping.

STEP 2: **Take your Measurements** (page 21)

Just focus on weight for now, but if you want to measure your waist and other areas, please do it today.

STEP 3: **Connect for Accountability**

Our Facebook Support Group is "My Weight Loss Community". It's not required but you will lose up to 2x's more weight if you have a group to work with, and it's part of the daily challenges to help you get amazing results. Don't worry this is optional, but it is good to have a support person/group during any of life's changes.

Okay, I know that was a lot of information. I also know anything new can seem very overwhelming at the beginning, it's okay; we have all been there. My goal is to help you get the results you are after and help you every step of the way, so you never feel alone in this process. Take a deep breath, and just take it one step at a time.

Once again, welcome! You have the potential to achieve amazing things and I am so excited and honored to be part of it.

If you've purchased the paper book, just email me proof of purchase and you'll get a login to access to 100s of more menus and bonus files (check your spam folder if you don't see it). EMAIL: Pam@3weekslimdownchallenge.com

Example Shopping list

Simple Shopping List

Fruits & Veggies

- Oranges   4
- Apples   6
- Strawberries   3lbs
- Tomatoes   1lb
- Lettuce   1 bag
- Spinach   1 bag

Veggies

- Celery   1 bunch
- Asparagus   14oz
- Potatoes (5 white, 2 sweet)
- Green Beans 12oz bag
- Broccoli   2-12oz bags
- Cauliflower 2-12oz bags

Meats

- Tilapia   16 oz
- Chicken   16oz
- Sirloin Steak   7oz
- Lean Beef   7oz
- Shrimp   7oz

Snacks

- Hamburger buns bag
- Skim Milk   1/2 gal.
- Eggs   1/2 doz.
- Instant Oatmeal   box

Example 7 Day Menu Plan, with 150 flex calories daily

Day 1:	115 0 total calories	Cal.	Day 2:	1137 total calories	Cal.
Breakfast	Orange, Coffee, & Oatmeal	199	Breakfast	Apple, Coffee, & Hard Boiled Egg	152
Snacks	Apple, & yogurt	302	Snacks	Strawberries(6oz) &	175
Lunch	Chicken (3 oz)	87	Lunch	Hamburger (3 oz) w/bun tomato & lettuce	300
Lunch Side	Baked Potato & Spinach (6oz)	135	Lunch Side	Cauliflower (6oz)	40
Lunch Side	green beans (6oz)	35	Lunch Side	Strawberries (6-7)	80
Dinner	Tilapia (3.5oz)	100	Dinner	Shrimp (3.5oz)	100
Dinner Sides	Broccoli (6oz) & 8oz milk	142	Dinner Side	Asparagus (7oz) & Baked Sweet Potato	140
Snack	Your favorite snack	150	Snack	Your favorite snack	150

Day 3 & 5:	1132 total calories	Cal.	Day 4:	1104 total calories	Cal.
Breakfast	Orange, Coffee, & yogurt	169	Breakfast	Strawberries, Coffee, & Oatmeal	175
Snacks	Apple, & 2 Boiled Eggs	272	Snacks	Apple, & yogurt	302
Lunch	Chicken (3 oz)	87	Lunch	Sirloin Steak (3.5oz)	150
Lunch Side	Broccoli (6oz) & 8oz milk	140	Lunch Side	Baked Sweet Potato	100
Lunch Side	Baked Potato	100	Lunch Side	Orange	80
Dinner	Tilapia (3.5oz)	100	Dinner	Chicken (3 oz)	87
Dinner Sides	Green beans & Cauliflower(6oz)	75	Dinner Side	Green beans & celery	60
Snack	Favorite snack & Strawberries (6-7)	195	Snack	Your favorite snack	150

Day 6:	1163 total calories	Cal.	Day 7	1117 total calories	Cal.
Breakfast	Strawberries (6-7), Coffee, & Yogurt	145	Breakfast	Coffee & Apple	72
Snacks	Wheat thins (16) & Orange	199	Snacks	Orange & Yogurt	230
Lunch	Sirloin Steak (3.5oz) & Lettuce	160	Lunch	Hamburger (3 oz) w/bun tomato & lettuce	300
Lunch Side	Broccoli (6oz)	140	Lunch Side	Cauliflower (6oz)	40
Lunch Side	Green beans & Tomatoes (7oz)	75	Lunch Side	Strawberries	45
Dinner	Tilapia (3.5oz) & 8oz milk	174	Dinner	Shrimp (6oz)	180
Dinner Sides	Asparagus (7oz) & 1/2 can soup	120	Dinner Side	Baked Potato	100
Snack	Favorite snack	150	Snack	Your favorite snack	150

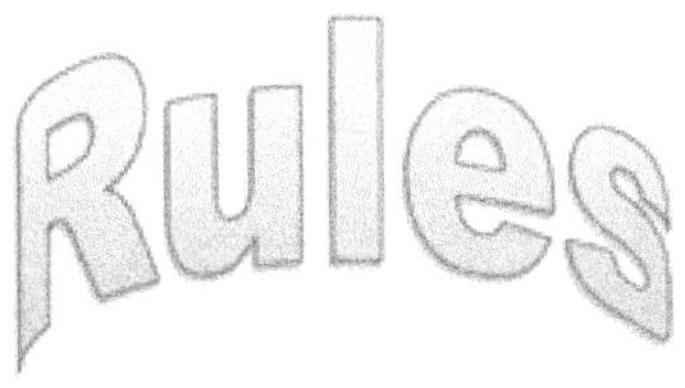

1. Have fun, don't think of what you can't do. Think of what you can, and how the results will make you feel.

2. Drinks lots of water. It keeps you full, hydrated, and cleanses the body.

3. Stay positive, don't worry about a set-back, just start over the next day.

4. Stick to foods you like. If you like chicken more than fish, just exchange equal calories. If you like chocolate (a little goes a long way) just switch out an equal calorie side item or snack. As long as you are eating the same number of calories it's more important to enjoy your day, than stick to an inflexible plan.

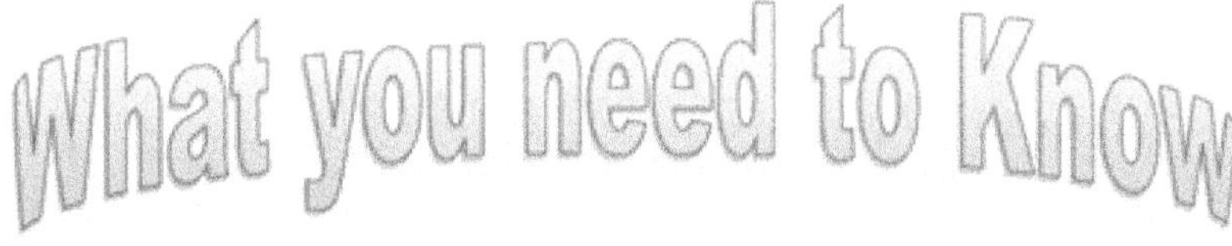

1. Know your starting weight and be honest of where you are.

2. Know your realistic healthy goal weight for your age & height. Hint: It is probably is not what you weighed in high school.

3. You need to know how many calories a day you typically burn based on your activity.

4. Know that it takes burning an extra ~3500 calories to burn off a pound of fat.

5. You need to understand losing weight is 80% what you eat. Get that right first, before doing any exercise program. Tip : Write down your food intake.

6. Understand: If you are a 40 year old 5'6" female and weigh 160 pounds, you burn ~2000 calories with normal activity. If you eat ~1200 calories/day for a week (800x7=5600, 5600/3500=1.6) you are guaranteed to lose wieght.

Weight Loss Math (to lose more than 1 pound a week):
2000-1200 = 800 daily calorie defecate x 7 days = 2600 calories burned/ week

CHAPTER 6: DAY 1

--- Let's Get Started Right ---

Congratulations on starting Day 1 of your Challenge. The next 3 Weeks are going to be so exciting!

This book is here to give you the tools and the steps to get started on the right path. It cannot force you to be successful, but it can provide you with the tools that will help pave the way for your success. Your responsibility is to take these tools and make them unique to your style to lead a healthy and fulfilling life.

The hope is to prevent you from 're-inventing the wheel' by sharing what has worked with other individuals and me to get and stay healthy.

So, let's get started.

.

Today's Challenge

Have an Accountability Partner: Talk to a friend or use our FB Community. Be honest with someone, and answer these questions
- Which Menu are you starting with?
- Why did you decide to join this Challenge?
- What's one thing they can do to help you reach your goals?

Date____________

Today's Plan

<table>
<tr><td>

To Do/Goals:

- ○ __________________
- ○ __________________
- ○ __________________
- ○ __________________
- ○ __________________
- ○ __________________

</td><td>

Daily Good Habits

○ Vitamins

○ 7+ hours of sleep

○ Quiet Time

</td></tr>
</table>

Food Journal

	Food/Beverage	Calories
Breakfast		
Lunch		
Dinner		
Snacks		
	Total	

Fitness		**Min.**

Water Intake 8+ cups

○ ○ ○ ○ ○ ○ ○ ○

Notes

____

____

____

____

____

____

____

____

Improvement Ideas

____

____

____

Gratitude Journal
(5 things you are grateful for today)

1) _______________________________________

2) _______________________________________

3) _______________________________________

4) _______________________________________

5) _______________________________________

DAY 2

--- Let's Get Your Goals & House in Order ---

Setting goals are critical to achieving results, and can provide you with focus, motivation, and a means of measuring your progress.

Rewarding yourself is key! Plan a special activity or gift at incremental goals, don't wait for your end goal.

This next part is a real challenge!!

Take a good look at the foods in your house that you did not buy for this week.

What you eat accounts for most of your results. It's key to stick with your program's list, or at least the calories and healthy alternates, if you are switching up a few items.

Look around your home and spend some time today throwing out (or giving away) as many of the unhealthy foods and beverages from your refrigerator and pantry that you can stand to. The truth is, if the "treat" isn't around when you're craving it, you CAN'T eat it. Chances are, your urges will pass long before you drive all the way to the store.

Today's Challenge

- What is your goal for this 3-Week Slim Down?
- What one item did you throw out (or gave way)?

Date____________

Today's Plan

To Do/Goals:

- ○ ____________________
- ○ ____________________
- ○ ____________________
- ○ ____________________
- ○ ____________________
- ○ ____________________

Daily Good Habits

○ Vitamins

○ 7+ hours of sleep

○ Quiet Time

Food Journal

	Food/Beverage	Calories
Breakfast		
Lunch		
Dinner		
Snacks		

Total	

Fitness		Min.

Water Intake 8+ cups

○ ○ ○ ○ ○ ○ ○ ○

Notes

____

____

____

____

____

____

____

Improvement Ideas

____

____

____

Gratitude Journal
(5 things you are grateful for today)

1) ____

2) ____

3) ____

4) ____

5) ____

DAY 3

--- Committed to your best every day! ---

Here are 3 tips to help you make the most of your hard work:

1.	Get plenty of sleep—at least 7 to 8 hours. Catching those z's is really-important to help your body recover and build muscle.

2.	Drink plenty of water! It's crucial to your weight loss. You might mistakenly think you are hungry when you are really dehydrated. Staying hydrated keeps your cardiovascular system running smoothly.

3.	Make sure you're getting the nutrition specific to your body, if you need fewer carbs, just switch out a potato for another apple or more meat.

Modification is a Positive Word

If your doctor recommends a specific instruction, listen.

Above all, listen to your body. This is your meal plan, to modify as needed. Hopefully, you already tossed all the junk from your home. Now for the fun part—shopping for healthy food! A shopping tip that makes a big difference is to stock your cart with at least 30% veggies!
Remember when I said listen to your body, well…… don't listen if it wants cake :-). It's really telling you it wants another apple.

Today's Challenge

- Rate on a scale of 1-10 (10 being the best) how you did with your water intake yesterday?
- Rate how well did you stick to your calories?

Date_____________

Today's Plan

To Do/Goals:

- ○ _______________________
- ○ _______________________
- ○ _______________________
- ○ _______________________
- ○ _______________________
- ○ _______________________

Daily Good Habits

○ Vitamins

○ 7+ hours of sleep

○ Quiet Time

Food Journal

	Food/Beverage	Calories
Breakfast		
Lunch		
Dinner		
Snacks		

Total	

Fitness		Min.

Water Intake 8+ cups

○ ○ ○ ○ ○ ○ ○ ○

Notes

____

____

____

____

____

____

____

____

Improvement Ideas

____

____

____

Gratitude Journal
(5 things you are grateful for today)

1) _______________________________________

2) _______________________________________

3) _______________________________________

4) _______________________________________

5) _______________________________________

DAY 4

--- Check-In ---

We're more than halfway through the first week!

How are you feeling so far?

If you're struggling at all, don't beat yourself up! I promise, your will power will get stronger.

Trust the process and believe in yourself — that's how you get results!

Focus on the reasons you started this.

Today's Challenge

Challenge Review (Catch-up)

In case missed any of the first 3 challenges, here they are. (either reply or post)

Day 1:
- Why are you doing this Challenge?

Day 2:
- What are your goals?
- What 'treat' did you remove from your home to help?

Day 3:
Rate on a scale of 1-10 (10 being the best) how you did on Water & Calories?

YOUR WATER AND FOOD INTAKE IS THAT IMPORTANT!

JUST SHOOT ME A NOTE AT
PAM@3WEEKSLIMDOWNCHALLENGE.COM
IF YOU HAVE ANY QUESTIONS.

Date_____________

Today's Plan

<table>
<tr><td>**To Do/Goals:**</td><td>**Daily Good Habits**</td></tr>
</table>

To Do/Goals:
- ○ _______________
- ○ _______________
- ○ _______________
- ○ _______________
- ○ _______________
- ○ _______________

Daily Good Habits

○ Vitamins

○ 7+ hours of sleep

○ Quiet Time

Food Journal

	Food/Beverage	Calories
Breakfast		
Lunch		
Dinner		
Snacks		
	Total	

Fitness		**Min.**

Water Intake 8+ cups

○ ○ ○ ○ ○ ○ ○ ○

Notes

____

____

____

____

____

____

____

____

Improvement Ideas

____

____

____

Gratitude Journal
(5 things you are grateful for today)

1) ____

2) ____

3) ____

4) ____

5) ____

DAY 5

--- Exercise ---

You don't need to exercise to lose weight. Totally true, but...

Exercise is still one of the best ways to maintain your health and accelerate your weight loss if you are on a healthy eating plan.

Food has to be #1, but once you have that down, get moving, in whatever way you can. Walking is the simplest and there is no need to buy equipment.

We are all at a different starting point so just do a little more today than you typically do.

Are you feeling at all sore or tired today?
If so, that's GOOD! It means your body is working. You're pushing your body in new ways, you're breaking down the fat, so it can burn. Sometimes when you are burning fat, it releases toxins into your body, which now can be flushed out. Don't worry, this will pass, and you will have more energy in a few days.

This also helps explain why you might be a little hungry, even if you've been following your nutrition plan. When your body is in fat burning mode, it starts craving more nutrients. Just let your body get those nutrients out of your stored fat cells, not from new food. It's all just part of the process of getting stronger and fitter!

Today's Challenge

- Get moving - Now, I mean right now!
- Go for a walk, do 10 jumping jacks or 5 push-ups before reading the next line. Maybe put in a workout DVD you have sitting out.

Date______________

Today's Plan

<table>
<tr><td>To Do/Goals:</td><td>Daily Good Habits</td></tr>
<tr><td>
○ ___________________
○ ___________________
○ ___________________
○ ___________________
○ ___________________
○ ___________________
</td><td>
○ Vitamins

○ 7+ hours of sleep

○ Quiet Time
</td></tr>
</table>

Food Journal

	Food/Beverage	Calories
Breakfast		
Lunch		
Dinner		
Snacks		

Total	

Fitness		**Min.**

Water Intake 8+ cups

○ ○ ○ ○ ○ ○ ○ ○

Notes

Improvement Ideas

Gratitude Journal
(5 things you are grateful for today)

1) _______________________________________

2) _______________________________________

3) _______________________________________

4) _______________________________________

5) _______________________________________

DAY 6

--- Nutrition Boost ---

Remember, every expert started their journey as a beginner. Don't be discouraged if things are tough right now; keep at it and you will see progress!

Today's nutrition boost comes from a very simple fruit. This should be your "go-to" food if you are feeling a bit hungry on your menu plan. I'm sure you've heard...

"An apple a day keeps the doctor away."

It has some truth. Each medium apple contains about 80 calories and five grams of dietary fiber, more than most cereals.

It also has phytonutrients, which along with the dietary fiber, has been shown to reduced risk of the following:
- heart disease, stroke, prostate cancer
- type 2 diabetes & asthma

Sources: Journal of Agricultural and Food Chemistry and lifescript.com

Today's Challenge

- How many times a week do you eat an apple? Can you commit to at least 3+?
- How do you like to eat your apples?
  - ✓ Natural
  - ✓ Sliced

******My favorite is sliced with cinnamon and sugar substitute
(warm up in the microwave for 30 seconds)
It's like apple pie, and only 80 calories.

Date____________

Today's Plan

<table>
<tr><td>**To Do/Goals:**</td><td>**Daily Good Habits**</td></tr>
</table>

- ○ ___________________
- ○ ___________________
- ○ ___________________
- ○ ___________________
- ○ ___________________
- ○ ___________________

○ Vitamins

○ 7+ hours of sleep

○ Quiet Time

Food Journal

	Food/Beverage	Calories
Breakfast		
Lunch		
Dinner		
Snacks		
	Total	

Fitness		**Min.**

Water Intake 8+ cups

○ ○ ○ ○ ○ ○ ○ ○

Notes

____

____

____

____

____

____

____

____

Improvement Ideas

____

____

____

Gratitude Journal
(5 things you are grateful for today)

1) ____

2) ____

3) ____

4) ____

5) ____

DAY 7

--- Week 1 is in the books! ---

Today is the last day of your first 7 days!! You are 1/3 through this challenge.

Congratulations!!

Hopefully, you are feeling a bit better, lighter, and stronger than a week ago.

Today is the day that you plan for next week. If you feel like the menu you started with is a little less or more calories than you want to go with next week, pick a new menu or repeat the same with a bit of adjustment.

You can follow this basic list, as a very general guide.

Current Weight	Suggested Menu Plan
140 or less	1000-1200 Calories
140-160	1100-1300 Calories
160-180	1200-1400 Calories
180-200	1300-1500 Calories....so on...

Need Help?

Email me at pam@3weekslimdownchallenge.com, and I will send you the one that is right for you if you need help.

Above all, listen to your body. This is your meal plan, to modify as needed. You will lose just as much weight if you add an apple or orange when you are hungry. If that doesn't make sense, I'll explain. It's because the fiber will keep you full and satisfied. If you are starving and miserable you will either quit or go for that candy bar. Just make sure you modify with healthy choices.

<u>Today's Challenge</u>

Now that you have 7 days of your challenge under your belt,
- What's one thing you want to do better next week?
- What menu plan are you shopping for next week?

Date____________

Today's Plan

To Do/Goals:

- ○ _______________
- ○ _______________
- ○ _______________
- ○ _______________
- ○ _______________
- ○ _______________

Daily Good Habits

○ Vitamins

○ 7+ hours of sleep

○ Quiet Time

Food Journal

	Food/Beverage	Calories
Breakfast		
Lunch		
Dinner		
Snacks		

Total	

Fitness		Min.

Water Intake 8+ cups

○ ○ ○ ○ ○ ○ ○ ○

Notes

____

____

____

____

____

____

____

Improvement Ideas

____

____

____

Gratitude Journal
(5 things you are grateful for today)

1) ____

2) ____

3) ____

4) ____

5) ____

DAY 8

--- Check-In / Motivation ---

"Motivation is what gets you started. Habit is what keeps you going." ~Jim Rohn

WEEK 2, here we go...

Did you see the scale drop last week?
I love, love, love to see people get success, so brag about it!

This is a new DAY, a new WEEK, don't get relaxed and backtrack.

If you modify your plan **don't** add in any of these:

Fast foods
Fried foods
Cookies
Candy
Cakes and other sweets
Frozen foods

Today's Challenge

Week 1: Weigh in time, how did you do?

Record your weight & measurements on page 120.

Date____________

Today's Plan

To Do/Goals:

- ○ ________________
- ○ ________________
- ○ ________________
- ○ ________________
- ○ ________________
- ○ ________________

Daily Good Habits

○ Vitamins

○ 7+ hours of sleep

○ Quiet Time

Food Journal

	Food/Beverage	Calories
Breakfast		
Lunch		
Dinner		
Snacks		
	Total	

Fitness		**Min.**

Water Intake 8+ cups

○ ○ ○ ○ ○ ○ ○ ○

Notes

____

____

____

____

____

____

____

____

Improvement Ideas

____

____

____

Gratitude Journal
(5 things you are grateful for today)

1) ____

2) ____

3) ____

4) ____

5) ____

DAY 9

--- Words to ponder ---

"Can it be a mistake that 'STRESSED' is 'DESSERTS' spelled backwards?"

I hope you are enjoying your menu plans. They are full of delicious foods, but do you ever wonder what is the best thing to have for dessert on a diet?

Here are several choices that you can switch with any of the foods on your plan to give yourself a Healthy Treat.

Berries
This is the perfect weight-loss food. Berries have natural fructose sugar that satisfies your longing for sweets and enough fiber, so you absorb fewer calories when you eat them. British researchers found that the high content of insoluble fiber in fruits reduces the absorption of calories from foods enough to promote weight loss without hampering nutrition.

Berries are a great source of potassium that can help with blood pressure control. Blackberries have about 74 calories per cup, blueberries 81, raspberries 60 and strawberries 45. So, use your imagination and enjoy the berry of your choice.

Melons
Now, here's great taste and great nutrition in a low-calorie package! One cup of cantaloupe balls has about 62 calories, one cup of honeydew balls has 62 calories and one cup of watermelon balls has only 49 calories. They have some of the highest fiber content of any food and are delicious. Throw in handsome quantities of vitamins A and C plus a whopping 547 mg of potassium in that cup of cantaloupe, and you have a fat-burning health food beyond compare.

Today's Challenge

What's your favorite Treat or Dessert that does not give you any guilt? Or make a list of more than one treat or dessert.

Date_____________

Today's Plan

<table>
<tr><td>

To Do/Goals:

</td><td>

Daily Good Habits

</td></tr>
</table>

- ○ _______________________
- ○ _______________________
- ○ _______________________
- ○ _______________________
- ○ _______________________
- ○ _______________________

○ Vitamins

○ 7+ hours of sleep

○ Quiet Time

Food Journal

	Food/Beverage	Calories
Breakfast		
Lunch		
Dinner		
Snacks		

	Total	

Fitness		Min.

Water Intake 8+ cups

○ ○ ○ ○ ○ ○ ○ ○

Notes

____

____

____

____

____

____

____

Improvement Ideas

____

____

____

Gratitude Journal
(5 things you are grateful for today)

1) ______________________________________

2) ______________________________________

3) ______________________________________

4) ______________________________________

5) ______________________________________

DAY 10

--- Focus on Health ---

Did you know some people actually GAIN weight before they start losing it? If you notice the scale has been creeping up, several things could be happening:

1. As crazy as it sounds, maybe you're not eating enough.

Make sure you don't shock your body too much by eating too little. We all like quick results but eating the right amount for your current size and activity level, is critical for healthy weight loss.

2. You might be retaining water due to muscle inflammation if you are working out.

This should subside as your body becomes accustomed to working out. Sometimes you can build muscle faster than dropping fat. This will switch fast in a few weeks.

3. Excess stress could also be the culprit.

Putting your body under too much stress by under-eating and performing a lot of high-intensity exercise that you're not used to could cause your body to release cortisol, which can add fat around your midsection. Don't give up! In a couple of weeks, these issues tend to resolve themselves. But if you're still having problems, I encourage you to ask questions and find answers.

Today's Challenge

- Rate how well you did on sticking to your calorie goals and water intake 1 through 10.
- Do one thing to relax today.

Date____________

Today's Plan

<table>
<tr><td>To Do/Goals:</td><td>Daily Good Habits</td></tr>
</table>

- ○ ____________________
- ○ ____________________
- ○ ____________________
- ○ ____________________
- ○ ____________________
- ○ ____________________

○ Vitamins

○ 7+ hours of sleep

○ Quiet Time

Food Journal

	Food/Beverage	Calories
Breakfast		
Lunch		
Dinner		
Snacks		
	Total	

Fitness		**Min.**

Water Intake 8+ cups

○ ○ ○ ○ ○ ○ ○ ○

Notes

____

____

____

____

____

____

____

____

Improvement Ideas

____

____

____

Gratitude Journal
(5 things you are grateful for today)

1) _______________________________________

2) _______________________________________

3) _______________________________________

4) _______________________________________

5) _______________________________________

DAY 11

--- Staying Motivated ---

"People often say that motivation doesn't last. Well, neither does bathing – that's why we recommend it daily."
~Zig Ziglar

It's so much easier to reach your goals when you know others are on the same journey. You're almost done with Week 2!

When I'm really down on myself, it's harder for me to stick to my plan, which makes it even harder to make any progress. Sound familiar? If you're finding it hard to stay consistent because you're feeling really stuck, and it seems like such a long journey. Encourage others, and it comes back around 10x's.

Helping others has totally helped me stay consistent by making me want to be better …make a note of how it works for you!

Today's Challenge

Reach out to someone from the FB Support Group at https://www.facebook.com/groups/myweightlosscommunity and give them some motivation for the day!

Or reach out to someone in person.

Date____________

Today's Plan

To Do/Goals:	Daily Good Habits

To Do/Goals:
- ○ ___________________
- ○ ___________________
- ○ ___________________
- ○ ___________________
- ○ ___________________
- ○ ___________________

Daily Good Habits
- ○ Vitamins
- ○ 7+ hours of sleep
- ○ Quiet Time

Food Journal

	Food/Beverage	Calories
Breakfast		
Lunch		
Dinner		
Snacks		
	Total	

Fitness		**Min.**

Water Intake 8+ cups

○ ○ ○ ○ ○ ○ ○ ○

Notes

____

____

____

____

____

____

____

____

Improvement Ideas

____

____

____

Gratitude Journal
(5 things you are grateful for today)

1) ____

2) ____

3) ____

4) ____

5) ____

DAY 12

--- Focus on Fitness ---

Too many people confine their exercise to:

- jumping to conclusions
- running up bills
- stretching the truth
- bending over backwards
- lying down on the job
- sidestepping responsibility
- pushing their luck

Any movement is better than making excuses as to why you can't.

You know what they say…it's easier to stick with it than to start over! I want you to focus on being consistent with your nutrition this week, and add in a bit of movement, too.

Sometime when you are dieting or just in general, we don't get all the nutrition we need from our food. If we eat foods high in fiber, it helps slow down your digestive process, which helps nutrient absorption.

Vitamins B12 and D are critical to blood flow and energy level. Make sure you are getting your day's recommended amount.

<u>Today's Challenge</u>

- How do you stay on point with your nutrition?
- Do you prep your meals for the week?
- Write notes on what you are doing to stay consistent!

Date____________

Today's Plan

To Do/Goals:	Daily Good Habits

To Do/Goals:
- ○ ______________________
- ○ ______________________
- ○ ______________________
- ○ ______________________
- ○ ______________________
- ○ ______________________

Daily Good Habits
- ○ Vitamins
- ○ 7+ hours of sleep
- ○ Quiet Time

Food Journal

	Food/Beverage	Calories
Breakfast		
Lunch		
Dinner		
Snacks		
	Total	

Fitness		Min.

Water Intake 8+ cups

○ ○ ○ ○ ○ ○ ○ ○

Notes

____

____

____

____

____

____

____

Improvement Ideas

____

____

____

Gratitude Journal
(5 things you are grateful for today)

1) _______________________________________

2) _______________________________________

3) _______________________________________

4) _______________________________________

5) _______________________________________

DAY 13

--- Focus on Nutrition ---

"Our food should be our medicine and our medicine should be our food." ~Hippocrates

I don't know about you, but I find it easy to overeat at mealtime. What can I say, I just LOVE food!

To avoid feeling stuffed, portion out your meal, eat it and then wait for 20–30 minutes for your brain to tell if your body is full. This trick usually works and helps keep your nutrition on track.

Healthy Eating Plate

Forget that old food pyramid you grew up with. Think:

- 30% meat
- 30% Starch
- 40% Veggies

Best Tip: Drink a full glass of water, before you start eating, and finish a 2nd glass halfway through your meal.

Today's Challenge

- Do you have any tips to avoid overeating?
- Write them down.

Date____________

Today's Plan

To Do/Goals:

- ○ _______________________
- ○ _______________________
- ○ _______________________
- ○ _______________________
- ○ _______________________
- ○ _______________________

Daily Good Habits

○ Vitamins

○ 7+ hours of sleep

○ Quiet Time

Food Journal

	Food/Beverage	Calories
Breakfast		
Lunch		
Dinner		
Snacks		

Total	

Fitness		**Min.**

Water Intake 8+ cups

○ ○ ○ ○ ○ ○ ○ ○

Notes

Improvement Ideas

Gratitude Journal
(5 things you are grateful for today)

1)

2)

3)

4)

5)

DAY 14

--- Relaxation ---

Remember, stress releases cortisol, which can make it harder to lose fat from your midsection.

Unfortunately, the negative effects of stress don't stop there. It can also impair recovery and muscle function for up to 96 hours after a tough workout—NOT COOL. That's why it's important to step back and take a deep breath every once in a while.

Studies show that even sitting quietly and focusing on your breathing for just 10 minutes a day can reduce psychological stress by up to 44%.

Here's one reason to catch more z's at night, to help you get weight loss results!

Not only is it important to lock in those 8 hours of sleep each night to help your body recover from your day, but a good night's rest can actually help with muscle growth. If you are starting to move more, your muscles are getting stronger, and sleep assists every part of getting healthier.

Today's Challenge

- Find some quite time today, just 2 minutes can make a big difference.

Date____________

Today's Plan

To Do/Goals:	Daily Good Habits

To Do/Goals:
- ○ ____________________
- ○ ____________________
- ○ ____________________
- ○ ____________________
- ○ ____________________
- ○ ____________________

Daily Good Habits
- ○ Vitamins
- ○ 7+ hours of sleep
- ○ Quiet Time

Food Journal

	Food/Beverage	Calories
Breakfast		
Lunch		
Dinner		
Snacks		
	Total	

Fitness		**Min.**

Water Intake 8+ cups

○ ○ ○ ○ ○ ○ ○ ○

Notes

____

____

____

____

____

____

____

____

Improvement Ideas

____

____

____

Gratitude Journal
(5 things you are grateful for today)

1) _______________________________________

2) _______________________________________

3) _______________________________________

4) _______________________________________

5) _______________________________________

DAY 15

--- Check-In ---

"There are no secrets to success. It is the result of preparation, hard work, and learning from failure."
~Colin Powell

Congrats!

You made it to Week 3.

How are you feeling?

If you ever have any questions, feel free to send them my way and together we will find a solution that works for you.

Just never Quit!

Today's Challenge

Week 2: Weigh in time, how did you do?

Record your weight & measurements on page 120.

Date______________

Today's Plan

To Do/Goals:

- ○ _______________________
- ○ _______________________
- ○ _______________________
- ○ _______________________
- ○ _______________________
- ○ _______________________

Daily Good Habits

○ Vitamins

○ 7+ hours of sleep

○ Quiet Time

Food Journal

	Food/Beverage	Calories
Breakfast		
Lunch		
Dinner		
Snacks		

Total	

Fitness		Min.

Water Intake 8+ cups

○ ○ ○ ○ ○ ○ ○ ○

Notes

____

____

____

____

____

____

____

Improvement Ideas

____

____

____

Gratitude Journal
(5 things you are grateful for today)

1) ____

2) ____

3) ____

4) ____

5) ____

DAY 16

--- Health ---

Who needs the scale?

There are better ways to track your progress during your challenge than your weight. Really notice how your clothes fit, if moving feels easier, that's success. Also, check your measurements, knowing that you are losing inches will feel amazing!

Focus on tracking your measurements WEEKLY. Don't weigh yourself again until the morning of day 22 of this challenge.

Not only will this help you see meaningful change (like inches lost or muscle gained), but it will help us figure out if we need to adjust your calorie intake.

"Take care of your body.
It's the only place you have to live."
~Jim Rohn

Today's Challenge

Stop weighing yourself more than once a week.

- How often have you been weighing yourself?
- How hard will it be, to not weigh yourself for the next 5 days?

Date____________

Today's Plan

To Do/Goals:

- ○ _______________
- ○ _______________
- ○ _______________
- ○ _______________
- ○ _______________
- ○ _______________

Daily Good Habits

○ Vitamins

○ 7+ hours of sleep

○ Quiet Time

Food Journal

	Food/Beverage	Calories
Breakfast		
Lunch		
Dinner		
Snacks		

Total	

Fitness		Min.

Water Intake 8+ cups

○ ○ ○ ○ ○ ○ ○ ○

Notes

____

____

____

____

____

____

____

Improvement Ideas

____

____

____

Gratitude Journal
(5 things you are grateful for today)

1) ____

2) ____

3) ____

4) ____

5) ____

DAY 17

--- Focus on Nutrition ---

"If food is your best friend, it's also your worst enemy."
~Edward "Grandpa" Jones

I absolutely LOVE cereal and I have a feeling you might too.

Unfortunately, some cereals—even "healthy" ones—contain a ton of hidden sugars. So, make sure you read the labels and choose ones with a low-sugar content (5 grams or less), plenty of whole grains, and few (or no) extra preservatives.

If you really need to add a sweet kick to your morning bowl, just add some fruit!

Meal Prep Tip

Have you tried using mason jars for meal prep?

These are great for salads for the week because they keep the ingredients fresh, if you layer them properly. Then when you're ready to eat, all you have to do is shake 'em up!
Here are a few tips for creating the perfect, long-lasting mason jar salad:
Pour dressing in the bottom. That way your veggies stay crunchy and fresh.
Layer heartier ingredients like carrots or beans after the dressing. Pack your greens on top.

Today's Challenge

Break a bad habit

- What bad habits have you broken so far?
- Do you have any you can't seem to drop?

Date________________

Today's Plan

To Do/Goals:

- ○ __________________
- ○ __________________
- ○ __________________
- ○ __________________
- ○ __________________
- ○ __________________

Daily Good Habits

○ Vitamins

○ 7+ hours of sleep

○ Quiet Time

Food Journal

	Food/Beverage	Calories
Breakfast		
Lunch		
Dinner		
Snacks		
	Total	

Fitness		Min.

Water Intake 8+ cups

○ ○ ○ ○ ○ ○ ○ ○

Notes

____

____

____

____

____

____

____

Improvement Ideas

____

____

____

Gratitude Journal
(5 things you are grateful for today)

1) _______________________________________

2) _______________________________________

3) _______________________________________

4) _______________________________________

5) _______________________________________

DAY 18

--- Motivation Focused ---

"Act as if everything you do makes a difference. It does."
~William James

Don't feel like doing your best today? Instead of focusing on losing weight or getting "thinner," try focusing on how being healthier will increase your quality of life.

The effort you put in today can improve your mood and help you become stronger and more confident. That might be just the push you need to do something outside of your comfort zone!

We all unwind in different ways (confession: my favorite way to unwind is with popcorn and a movie). At least I try to stick with light popcorn.

Have you ever tried meditation? It's amazing to discover great new "non-food "pleasures in life.

Taking a few minutes out of your day to relax and reflect on your thoughts can do wonders for your mind, body, and stress levels. Here are a few things to keep in mind when learning how to meditate:

- Maintain a straight spine while sitting cross-legged in a chair or on the floor.
- Focus on your breathing—in through the nose and out through the mouth.
- Focus on something that makes you happy!

And don't worry if you get distracted—focus is like a muscle and meditation will help strengthen it!

Today's Challenge

- Find a new non-food Pleasure/Reward.
- What do you enjoy that fills your spirit?

Date_______________

Today's Plan

<table>
<tr><td>To Do/Goals:</td><td>Daily Good Habits</td></tr>
</table>

To Do/Goals:
- ○ _______________________
- ○ _______________________
- ○ _______________________
- ○ _______________________
- ○ _______________________
- ○ _______________________

Daily Good Habits
- ○ Vitamins
- ○ 7+ hours of sleep
- ○ Quiet Time

Food Journal

	Food/Beverage	Calories
Breakfast		
Lunch		
Dinner		
Snacks		
	Total	

Fitness		**Min.**

Water Intake 8+ cups

○ ○ ○ ○ ○ ○ ○ ○

Notes

____

____

____

____

____

____

____

Improvement Ideas

____

____

____

Gratitude Journal
(5 things you are grateful for today)

1) ______________________________

2) ______________________________

3) ______________________________

4) ______________________________

5) ______________________________

DAY 19

--- Focus on Fitness ---

Remember, the road to getting healthy and fit is a journey. It won't always be easy. There will come a day when you lack the motivation to get in more activity.

If that feeling persists, you might be in burnout mode. Don't worry—it doesn't have to last forever.

Find the shift. Inches will start melting off and you'll begin to feel better about yourself.

Your self-esteem will rise, and people will start to notice the difference in how happy and confident you are.

We're nearly done with this 3 Week program! Amazing, right? Think for a moment about when you started. If you want, share some of the lifestyle changes you've made since then and write them down.

<u>Today's Challenge</u>

- What are some foods/beverages you gave up?
- Is following the program as hard as you thought?
- Are there some delicious foods you're eating that you never thought you would?

Date____________

Today's Plan

<table>
<tr><td>To Do/Goals:</td><td>Daily Good Habits</td></tr>
</table>

To Do/Goals:
- ○ ____________________
- ○ ____________________
- ○ ____________________
- ○ ____________________
- ○ ____________________
- ○ ____________________

Daily Good Habits
- ○ Vitamins
- ○ 7+ hours of sleep
- ○ Quiet Time

Food Journal

	Food/Beverage	Calories
Breakfast		
Lunch		
Dinner		
Snacks		
	Total	

Fitness		Min.

Water Intake 8+ cups

○ ○ ○ ○ ○ ○ ○ ○

Notes

____

____

____

____

____

____

____

____

Improvement Ideas

____

____

____

Gratitude Journal
(5 things you are grateful for today)

1) _________________________________

2) _________________________________

3) _________________________________

4) _________________________________

5) _________________________________

DAY 20

--- One Day Left!! ---

You've got one day left in your challenge and I'm curious…has it positively impacted your life?

What changed? And what's next? Don't forget, this is NOT the end. Make those healthy habits we talked about a daily commitment and you'll continue to become the very best version of yourself!

Now that we're in the home stretch, you're probably thinking, "What's next?" or "How do I get even better results?"

You've got tons of options.

You could redo the challenge and maybe bump up to the next eating plan to build more lean muscle. Another option is to try a "hybrid" version of the challenge - one that combines what you've just completed with another challenge.

You can find more on our website. at https://www.removemyweight.com . If you want something completely different, we can find you a new program to challenge your health and fitness in a brand-new way.

Today's Challenge

- What changed?
- What's next?

Do you want a Do-Over? Email me at pam@3weekslimdownchallenge.com to get the online challenge or grab another book.

Date____________

Today's Plan

<table>
<tr><td>

To Do/Goals:

- ○ _______________
- ○ _______________
- ○ _______________
- ○ _______________
- ○ _______________
- ○ _______________

</td><td>

Daily Good Habits

○ Vitamins

○ 7+ hours of sleep

○ Quiet Time

</td></tr>
</table>

Food Journal

	Food/Beverage	Calories
Breakfast		
Lunch		
Dinner		
Snacks		

	Total	

Fitness		**Min.**

Water Intake 8+ cups

○ ○ ○ ○ ○ ○ ○ ○

Notes

____

____

____

____

____

____

____

____

Improvement Ideas

____

____

____

Gratitude Journal
(5 things you are grateful for today)

1) ____

2) ____

3) ____

4) ____

5) ____

DAY 21

--- Last Day ---

Don't stop today!

We're on the Last Day of the challenge. It's not over until the end of the day.

Don't check your weight until tomorrow morning.

Hopefully, you've developed a bunch of new habits that will help you continue living a healthier life. Track your food and finish strong today.

How excited are you? Over the past few weeks, I know you've conquered your doubts and arose to numerous challenges. It's been so inspiring and I'm glad to have been a part of it. You might be wondering if you can help others experience the same sense of empowerment. Your story and your success in life can inspire others, so be bold and brag about it.

Today's Challenge

- Write down how you FEEL (without checking the scale).

Date____________

Today's Plan

<table>
<tr><td>To Do/Goals:</td><td>Daily Good Habits</td></tr>
</table>

To Do/Goals:

- ○ ____________________
- ○ ____________________
- ○ ____________________
- ○ ____________________
- ○ ____________________
- ○ ____________________

Daily Good Habits

- ○ Vitamins
- ○ 7+ hours of sleep
- ○ Quiet Time

Food Journal

	Food/Beverage	Calories
Breakfast		
Lunch		
Dinner		
Snacks		

Total	

Fitness		Min.

Water Intake 8+ cups

○ ○ ○ ○ ○ ○ ○ ○

Notes

____

____

____

____

____

____

____

____

WRAP-UP
CONGRATULATIONS! YOU MADE IT!

You've successfully completed your challenge.
What an incredible accomplishment!
Remember to take your "after" weight, and measurements,
so you can compare your results to where you started 3
Weeks ago.

Gratitude Journal
(5 things you are grateful for today)

1) _______________________________________

2) _______________________________________

3) _______________________________________

4) _______________________________________

5) _______________________________________

CHAPTER 7: POST- SURVEY

Date __________

Who shops for food at your home?

____

Who prepares it? _______________________

What do you drink during the day?

____

What kind of meat do you usually buy?

___ beef, steak, pork chops   ___ chicken, turkey, fish

If you don't eat meat, what types of protein do you buy?

____

What type of meal or meals do you prepare most often?

___ fry   ___ bake   ___ broil   ___ slow cook   ___ grill

How many times a day do you eat?

____

What do you usually eat?

____

How many times do you **eat out** during the week?

____

What restaurant do you go to most often?

____

List any vitamins or dietary supplements you take here. How many of each do you take? How often?

____

If you eat any special foods for health or personal reasons, list what kind and how much

____

List any other medication you take prescription or over the counter. How many of each do you take? How often?

____

Do you full well rested and excited for the day, if not how often?

____

How healthy do you feel?

____

Do you feel optimistic about the next month? If so why?

____

Survey: Your Typical Servings in a Week

Dairy

_____ glass(es) (8 ounces) of whole milk

_____ glass(es) of 2% milk or 1% or skim milk

_____ 1 ounce slice(s) of cheese

_____ serving(s) of yogurt or cottage cheese

Vegetables

_____ scoop-sized helping(s) of vegetables

_____ small vegetable salad(s)

_____ medium-sized potato(es)

Fruits

_____ piece(s) of fruit (an apple, orange, banana, slice of melon, etc.)

_____ 1/2 cup(s) cooked or canned fruit

Meat

_____ small piece(s) of meat, fish, or poultry (about the size of a deck of cards)

_____ 2 eggs

_____ 1 cup(s) cooked dried beans or peas

_____ 4 tablespoons peanut butter

_______ **This page totals**

<u>Grains</u>

_____ slice(s) of bread or tortilla(s)

_____ small roll(s), biscuit(s), or muffin(s)

_____ 1/2 bun(s), English muffin(s), or bagel(s)

_____ cooked cereal, rice, or pasta

_____ small bowl(s) of cold cereal

<u>Sweets and Fats</u>

_____ 10 chips or french fries

_____ candy bar(s) or 3 small cookies

_____ slice(s) of pie or cake

_____ sweet roll(s) or donut(s)

_____ 1/2 cup(s) of ice cream

_____ rounded teaspoon(s) of margarine or butter

_____ tablespoon(s) of salad dressing

_____ Pizza, spaghetti, lasagna, or Mac and Cheese

<u>Drinks</u>

_____ 12-ounce soda drinks

_____ glass(es) of Kool-Aid or fruit punch

_____ energy drinks

_____ 12-ounce beer(s)

_____ 4 ounces of wine (small glass)

_____ shot(s) of liquor

_____ **This page totals**

Weigh-In

Measurements

Measurement	Body Fat %	Upper Chest	Chest	Waist	Stomach	Hips	Left Upper Arm	Right Upper Arm	Right Thigh	Left Thigh	Right Calf	Left Calf			
Start															
7 days															
14 days															
21 days															

Final Notes

CHAPTER 8: 25 FREE FOODS

Here is a list of foods that you don't have to count. It is great to have standby snacks and options to not worry about writing down. Now with that said, these are not calorie free, but they are low enough in calories that they are great go to items for those mid-day cravings.

Snacks that you don't have to Count!!

Many vegetables that are high in water and fiber content end up being "free" or "almost free." So, if you're in the mood for something with crunch, think about these "free" options ("Free" foods, eaten in reasonable quantities, don't have to be journaled):

1. 2 large celery stalks = 13 calories, 1.2 grams fiber

2. 2 cups shredded lettuce = 18 calories, 1.4 grams fiber

3. 1/2 cucumber = 20 calories, 1 gram fiber

4. 1 medium tomato = 25 calories, 1.3 grams fiber

5. 1/2 cup sugar snap peas = 30 calories, 3.4 grams fiber

6. 1 carrot = 30 calories, 2 grams fiber

7. cup jicama sticks = 45 calories, 6 grams fiber

8. 1 peach = 37 calories, 1.6 grams fiber

9. 1/2 grapefruit = 37 calories, 1.7 grams fiber

10. 1 cup sliced strawberries = 50 calories, 2.5 grams fiber

11. 1 cup watermelon pieces = 51 calories, 0.4 grams fiber

12. 1 cup papaya pieces = 54 calories, 2.5 grams fiber

13. 3/4 cup apricot halves = 55 calories, 2 grams fiber

14. 1 cup cantaloupe cubes = 56 calories, 1.3 grams fiber

15. 1 orange = 60 calories, 2.3 grams fiber

16. 1 cup winter mix vegetables = 25 calories, 2 grams fiber

17. 1 cup Tuscan-style vegetables = 25 calories, 2 grams fiber

18. 1 cup mixed broccoli, cauliflower, and carrots = 25 calories

19. 3/4 cup whole green beans = 25 calories, 2 grams fiber

20. 1/2 cup of Sugar-Free Jell-O = 10 calories

21. 94% fat-free microwave popcorn. 2 cups popped = 40 calories

22. Quaker Rice Snacks, Apple Cinnamon. 8 mini cakes = 60 calories

23. Quaker Rice Snacks, Caramel Corn. 8 mini cakes = 60 calories

24. Dreyer's Whole Fruit Bars, No Sugar Added (strawberry, tangerine, and raspberry). 1 bar = 30 calories, 1-gram fiber.

25. Dole Fruit Juice Bars, No Sugar Added (strawberry, grape, and raspberry). 1 pop = 30 calories

In addition to these "FREE" foods, you may add the follow condiments as much as you like.

Among spices as well as condiments, you can consume:

- Yellow mustard

- Horseradish

- Hot sauce

- Worcestershire sauce

- Salad dressings with fewer than 45 calories per tablespoon (tbsp)

Among herbs and spices you can consume:

- Basil
- Parsley
- Rosemary
- Thyme
- Chili powder
- Cumin
- Cinnamon
- Lemon
- Salt
- Pepper
- Cilantro
- Oregano
- Sage

Among sweeteners, these are recommended, if needed.

- Stevia

- Erythritol

Other items:

- Lemon Juice

- Garlic

- Salt-Free Seasoning Blends

- Basil

- Parsley

- Vegetable Broth

- Fresh Ginger

- Sautéed Onions and Garlic

- Flavored Vinegar

- Tea

- Instant Coffee and Espresso Powder

CHAPTER 9: 100 FOOD EXCHANGES

This Challenge is intended to simplify eating healthy not over complicate it. Therefore, you can eat anything from the list below in exchange for anything on any of the example menus. There are literally 100s of foods that you can eat.

The only thing not allowed for an exchange is highly processed or sugary snacks, like a Snickers. Basically, if it is a natural food in its original form, please enjoy it. If you are concerned about the exchange calories, use one of the many online apps such as "My Fitness Pal" or "Lose It". They have a database of 1000s of foods and are even more accurate than the estimates in this book.

Protein: Exchange for 3-4 ounces in any category

- Poultry items like Duck, Turkey, Chicken (skin off)
- Pork items
- Beef (lean portions)
- Fish items like Salmon, trout, cord, catfish, Shrimp
- Shellfish like oysters, mussels, lobster
- Organ meats like heart, liver, kidney
- Egg
- Lamb
- Goat

Fruits:

Apple
Apricot
Banana
Blackberry
Blueberry
Cantaloupe
Cherry
Cranberry
Date
Fig
Grape
Grapefruit
Honeydew
Kiwi
Lemon
Lime
Mango
Melon
Nectarine
Orange
Clementine
Peach
Pear
Plum
Prune (dried plum)

Pineapple

Pomegranate

Raspberry

Strawberry

Tangerine

Watermelon

Papaya

Passionfruit

Surprisingly the below list are fruits according to the scientific definition, but are also considered to be vegetables:

Avocado (substitute ½ weight)

Corn

Cucumber

Eggplant

Olive

Pea

Pumpkin

squash

Tomato

Zucchini

Vegetables:

acorn squash

alfalfa sprouts

artichoke

arugula

asparagus

banana squash

beansprouts

Beets

Bell pepper

black beans

black-eyed peas

bok choy

broccoli

brussels sprouts

butternut squash

cabbage

carrot

cauliflower

celery

chickpeas

chili pepper

Chives

Collard greens

corn

cucumber

eggplant

green beans

kale

kidney beans

Leek

lentils

lettuce

lima bean

mushrooms

navy beans

okra

onion

peas

pinto beans

pumpkin

quinoa

radish

rhubarb

soy beans

spaghetti squash

spinach

split peas

sweet potato

tomato

turnip

water chestnut

white potato

yam

CHAPTER 10: EXAMPLE MENUS

These examples are provided as a guide and can be followed exactly, but you may need to add calories to ensure that you are losing weight at a safe and steady pace for your current body. These menus are intended to be your base nutrient and are low enough that you don't have to worry about eating 4 oz instead of 3 oz, if you don't weigh your food exactly.

We are also going for simplicity, so they may include items that are not exactly following a plan strictly like a vegetarian or Paleo. Please follow the 80/20 rule. Eat healthy 80% of the time but give yourself a break so that you can still enjoy life. Be 20% flexible with imperfect dieting. With that said, don't eat more than 20% junk calories in a day, or you will be frustrated with your results.

Calorie amounts are approximate, since your cooking method and the store that the items are purchased at can cause them to be higher or lower. These menus are made to be cut or torn out of this book and taken to the store or posted where you need.

Most people find that is it easiest to eat every few hours. As an example:

- 8am Breakfast

- 10am Snack

- 12pm Lunch

- 2 pm Snack

- 4 pm Water (or light snack)

- 6 pm Dinner

- 8 pm Snack

This example is for someone on a day schedule. You may need to adjust based on your normal day or work schedule. In general, I've found that it is good to only be eating about 12 or less hours in the day. We are awake about 16 hours a day, but typically we don't need to eat much in the last 4 hours before bed. So only having a small snack after dinner is a recommend.

Higher Protein Week Example

Meal	Foods	Est. Calories
Day 1		1523
Morning	Ham, 3 slices (2 oz)	69
Morning	2 Eggs, cooked, Hard Boiled	144
Snack	**Yogurt, Greek, (6oz)**	100
Lunch	Beef, steaks, chopped (6oz)	526
Lunch	Cheese, cream, (1 tbsp)	19
Lunch	Turkey, 3 slices,	81
Snack	**Shrimp, cooked (6oz)**	168
Dinner	Bacon, cooked (2 slices)	108
Dinner	Pork, loin, trimmed (4 oz)	195
Dinner	Sour cream, (1 tbsp)	9
Snack	**Cheese, cottage, (1 cup)**	104
Day 2		1541
Morning	Bacon, cooked (2 slices)	108
Morning	2 Eggs, cooked, fried in olive oil	180
snack	**1cup red pepper &Asparagus 2cups**	110
Lunch	Fish, salmon (4 oz)	161
Lunch	Broccoli (2 cups) & Shrimp (6oz)	146
Lunch	Shrimp, cooked (3oz)	84
Lunch	Spinach, cooked, boiled (1 cup)	41
Snack	**Yogurt, Greek, non fat (6oz)**	106
Dinner	Beef, tenderloin (6 oz)	274
Dinner	Shrimp, cooked (6oz)	168
Dinner	Squash, zucchini (1 cup)	66
Dinner	Turkey, 3 slices,	81
Snack	**Celery (3-5" sticks)**	16
Day 3		1529
Morning	Bacon, cooked (2 slices)	108
Morning	2 Eggs, cooked, Hard Boiled	144
Snack	**Yogurt, Greek, (6oz)**	106
Lunch	Pork, loin, trimmed (4 oz)	195
Lunch	Cheese, cottage, (1 cup)	104
Lunch	Turkey, 3 slices,	81
Snack	**Shrimp, cooked (6oz)**	168
Dinner	Beef, steaks, chopped (6oz)	526
Dinner	Sour cream, (1 tbsp)	9
Dinner	Ham, 3 slices (2 oz)	69
Snack	**Cheese, cream, 1 tbsp**	19

Meal	Food	Est. Calories
Day 4		1420
Morning	Turkey, 3 slices,	81
Morning	2 Eggs, cooked, fried in olive oil	180
Snack	**Carrots, baby (16)**	70
Lunch	Beef, tenderloin 6oz &Broccoli 2cups	336
Lunch	Peppers, sweet, red (1 cup)	46
Lunch	Spinach, cooked, boiled (1 cup)	41
Lunch	Bacon, cooked (2 slices)	108
Snack	**Yogurt, Greek, (6oz)**	106
Dinner	Peppers, sweet, yellow (1 cup)	50
Dinner	Fish, salmon (4 oz)	161
Dinner	Asparagus (2 cups) & Shrimp (3oz)	148
Dinner	Squash, zucchini (1 cup)	66
Snack	**Cauliflower, raw (1 cup)**	27
Day 5 & 7		1499
Morning	Bacon, cooked (2 slices)	108
Morning	2 Eggs, cooked, Hard Boiled	144
Snack	**Yogurt, Greek, (6oz)**	106
Lunch	Beef, steaks, chopped (6oz)	526
Snack	**Shrimp, cooked (6oz)**	168
Dinner	Beef, tenderloin (6 oz)	274
Dinner	Ham, 3 slices (2 oz)	69
Snack	**Cheese, cottage, (1 cup)**	104
Day 6		1482
Morning	Bacon, cooked (2 slices)	108
Morning	2 Eggs, cooked, fried in olive oil	180
Snack	**Cheese, cottage, (1 cup)**	104
Snack	**Carrots, baby (16)**	70
Lunch	Broccoli (2 cups) & Salmon 4oz	223
Lunch	Spinach, cooked, boiled (1 cup)	41
Lunch	Turkey, 3 slices,	81
Snack	**Yogurt, Greek, (6oz)**	106
Dinner	Pork, loin, trimmed (4 oz)	195
Dinner	Cauliflower (2 cups) & Shrimp (6oz)	222
Dinner	Sour cream, (1 tbsp)	9
Dinner	Bacon, cooked (2 slices)	108
Snack	**Celery (3-5" sticks) & cream cheese**	35

Shopping List

Bacon (sugar free)	16 slices	Cheese, cream,	3 tbsp	Spinach, Frozen	3 cups
Eggs	14 large	Sour cream,	3 tablesp	Squash, zucchini	2 cups
Ham, sliced,	10 oz	Shrimp, cooked	42 oz	Peppers, sweet, red	2 pepper
Turkey, sliced,	15 slices	Yogurt, Greek,	42 oz	Peppers, sweet, yellow	1 pepper
Beef, tenderloin	4 fillets	Celery, raw	2 Stocks		
Beef, steak	24 oz	Carrots, baby	1 Bags		
Fish, salmon	12 oz	Asparagus	4 cups		
Pork, loin,	12 oz	Broccoli	6 cups		
Cheese, cottage,	5 cup	Cauliflower, raw	3 cups		

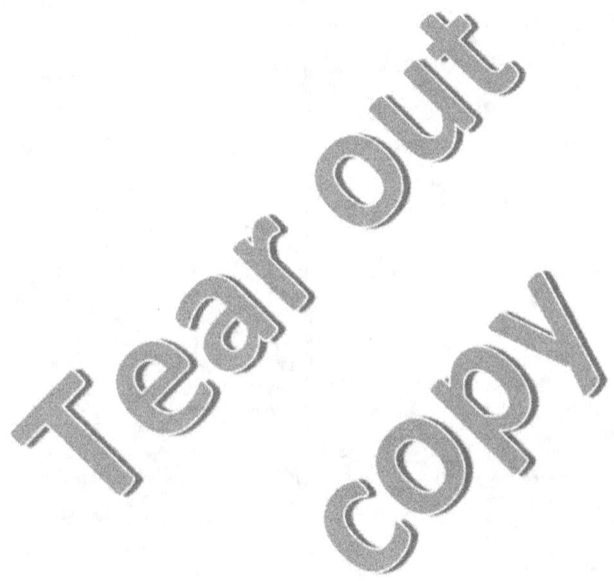

Low-Calorie Week Example

Day 1:	885 total calories	~Cal.
Breakfast	Orange & Coffee/Tea	70
Snack	Melba Toast (15 grams) ~3 pcs	60
Lunch	Grilled Chicken (4 oz)	130
Lunch Side	Spinach (6oz) & Yogurt	140
Lunch Side	Strawberries (6 oz. or 6-7)	45
Dinner	Tilapia (3.5oz)	100
Dinner Sides	Broccoli (6oz) & Baked Potato	170
Snack	Apple (medium) & Light Soup	170

Day 2:	885 total calories	~Cal.
Breakfast	Apple, Coffee/Tea	70
Snacks	Orange	70
Lunch	Hamburger (3 oz) 93% lean, no bun	150
Lunch Side	Cauliflower (6oz) & Light Soup	140
Lunch Side	Strawberries (6 oz)	45
Dinner	Shrimp (3.5oz)	110
Dinner Side	Asparagus (7oz) & Baked Potato	130
Snack	Tomatoes (7oz) & Yogurt	140

Day 3 & 5:	875 total calories	~Cal.
Breakfast	Orange, Coffee/Tea	70
Snacks	Melba Toast (10 grams) & yogurt	140
Lunch	Chicken (4 oz)	130
Lunch Side	Broccoli (6oz) & Potato	160
Lunch Side	Salad (no calorie dressing) & Apple	100
Dinner	Tilapia (3.5oz)	100
Dinner Sides	Cauliflower(6oz) & Light Soup	140
Snack	Strawberries (6-7)	45

Day 4:	845 total calories	~Cal.
Breakfast	Strawberries, Coffee/Tea	45
Snacks	Yogurt	100
Lunch	Sirloin Steak (3oz) & Potato	260
Lunch Side	Spinach Salad (no calorie dressing)	40
Lunch Side	Orange & Light soup	170
Dinner	Chicken (4 oz)	130
Dinner Side	Celery (7oz)	30
Snack	Apple (medium)	70

Day 6:	895 total calories	~Cal.
Breakfast	Strawberries (6-7), Coffee/Tea	45
Snacks	Orange	70
Lunch	Sirloin Steak (3oz)	160
Lunch Side	Cauliflower(6oz)	40
Lunch Side	Tomatoes (7oz) & Yougrt	140
Dinner	Tilapia (3.5oz) & Potato	200
Dinner Sides	Asparagus (7oz) & Melba Toast (10 g)	80
Snack	Apple & Light Soup	170

Day 7	875 total calories	~Cal.
Breakfast	Coffee/Tea & Apple	70
Snacks	Melba Toast (10 grams)	40
Lunch	Hamburger (3 oz) 93% lean, no bun	150
Lunch Side	Celery (7oz) & Light soup	130
Lunch Side	Strawberries 6 oz. or 6-7	45
Dinner	Shrimp (3.5oz)	110
Dinner Side	Broccoli (6oz) & Potato	160
Snack	Orange & Yogurt	170

Fruits & Veggies

- Oranges 7
- Apples 7
- Strawberries 3 lbs
- Tomatoes 2lb
- Lettuce 1 bag

Veggies

- Celery 1 bunch
- Asparagus 14oz
- Broccoli 2-12oz bags
- Cauliflower 2-12oz bags
- Spinach 1 bag
- Small Potatoes 1 bag

Meats

- Tilapia 14 oz
- Chicken 16oz
- Sirloin Steak 6oz
- Lean Beef 6oz
- Shrimp 7oz

Snacks

- Melba Toast 1box
- Tea packets 1box
- Coffee 1bag
- Yogurt 7
- Light Soup 4cans

****Light Soup would be one that is ~100 calories or less per serving.**

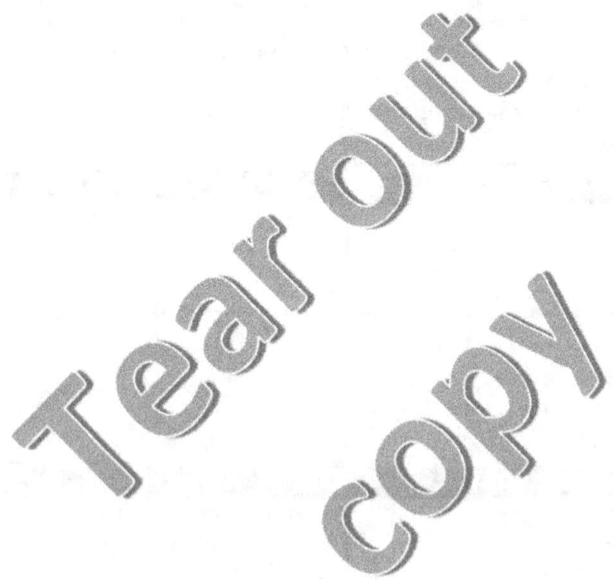

Simple Week Example

Meal	Foods	Est. Calories
Day 1		**1196**
Snack	Snacks, beef jerky, (1oz)	116
Morning	1 Hard Boiled Egg	72
Snack	Snacks, popcorn, microwave, low fat	120
Lunch	Chicken breast, mesquite (3oz)	102
Lunch	Asparagus (1 cup)	32
Lunch	Nonfat cottage cheese 1cup	104
Lunch	French fries (3 oz)	117
Lunch	Blackberries, raw 1 cup	62
Dinner	Fish, tilapia (3 oz) & Shrimp, cooked (	195
Dinner	Lettuce, 2 cups	20
Dinner	Dressing, fat-free	51
Dinner	Raspberries, raw 1 cup	64
Snack	Carrots, baby (8) & Yogurt (6oz)	141
Day 2		**1197**
Morning	2 Eggs, fried in olive oil	182
Snack	Nuts, almonds (~14)	85
Lunch	Pork, loin, trimmed (4 oz)	195
Lunch	Cauliflower (2 cups)	54
Lunch	Dressing, fat-free	51
Dinner	Lettuce, 2 cups	20
Lunch	Spinach, cooked (1 cup)	41
Snack	Carrots, baby (8)	35
Dinner	Turkey, 6 slices (4 oz)	190
Dinner	Broccoli (2 cups)	62
Dinner	White potato, baked (med)	114
Dinner	Blackberries, raw 1 cup	62
Snack	Yogurt (6oz)	106
Day 3		**1129**
Morning	Raspberries, raw 1 cup	64
Snack	Avocados, raw (.5 cup) & Yogurt (6oz	226
Morning	1 Hard Boiled Egg	72
Snack	Carrots, baby (8)	35
Lunch	Fish, tilapia (3 oz)	111
Lunch	Asparagus (1 cup) & Shrimp, cooked	116
Lunch	French fries (3 oz)	117
Lunch	Blackberries, raw 1 cup	62
Dinner	Chicken breast, mesquite (3oz)	102
Dinner	Nonfat cottage cheese 1cup	104
Snack	Snacks, popcorn, microwave, low fat	120

Meal	Food	Est. Calories
Day 4		**1183**
Morning	Blackberries, raw 1 cup	62
Morning	2 Eggs, Hard Boiled	144
Snack	Nuts, almonds (~14)	85
Lunch	Cauliflower (2 cups) & Turkey, 3 slice	135
Lunch	Lettuce, 2 cups	20
Lunch	Dressing, fat-free	51
Lunch	Raspberries, raw & Spinach, cooked (	105
Snack	Carrots, baby (8)	35
Snack	Snacks, beef jerky, (1oz)	116
Dinner	Pork, loin, trimmed (3 oz)	134
Dinner	Broccoli (2 cups)	62
Dinner	White potato, baked (med)	114
Snack	Snacks, popcorn, microwave, low fat	120
Day 5 & 7		**1118**
Morning	1 Hard Boiled Egg & Raspberries, raw	88
Snack	Carrots, baby (8)	35
Snack	Snacks, beef jerky, (1oz)	116
Lunch	Chicken breast, mesquite (3oz)	102
Lunch	Asparagus (1 cup)	32
Lunch	French fries (3 oz)	117
Lunch	Blackberries, raw 1 cup	62
Snack	Snacks, popcorn, microwave, low fat	120
Dinner	Broccoli (2 cups) & Turkey, 3 slices	143
Dinner	Nonfat cottage cheese 1cup	104
Dinner	White potato, baked (med)	114
Snack	Nuts, almonds (~14)	85
Day 6		**1111**
Morning	2 Eggs, Hard Boiled	144
Snack	Carrots, baby (8)	35
Lunch	Pork, loin, trimmed (3 oz)	134
Lunch	Cauliflower (2 cups)	54
Lunch	Shrimp, cooked (3oz)	84
Lunch	Blackberries, raw & Spinach, cooked	103
Snack	Avocados, raw (.5 cup) & Yogurt (6oz	226
Dinner	Fish, tilapia (3 oz)	111
Dinner	Lettuce, 2 cups	20
Dinner	Dressing, fat-free	51
Dinner	Raspberries, raw 1 cup	64
Snack	Nuts, almonds (~14)	85

Shopping List

Item	Qty	Item	Qty	Item	Qty
Eggs	10 large	Dressing, fat-free	8 tbsp	Avocados	1
Blackberries	7 cups	Shrimp, cooked	9 oz	Carrots, baby	2 Bags
Raspberries	6 cups	Yogurt, Greek, non fat	24 oz	Asparagus	4 cups
Turkey,low-fat, Sliced	6 oz	Nuts, almonds (~14)	3 oz	Broccoli	8 cups
Fish, tilapia	3 fillet	Snacks, beef jerky	4 oz	Cauliflower, raw	6 cups
Chicken Breast, mesquite,	12 ounce	Snacks, popcorn, microwav	5 oz	Lettuce	8 cups
Pork, loin,	10 oz	White potato, baked (med)	4 med.		
Turkey,low-fat, Sliced	4 oz	Frozen french fries	12 oz		
Cheese, cottage, nonfat	4 cup	Spinach, Frozen	3 cups		

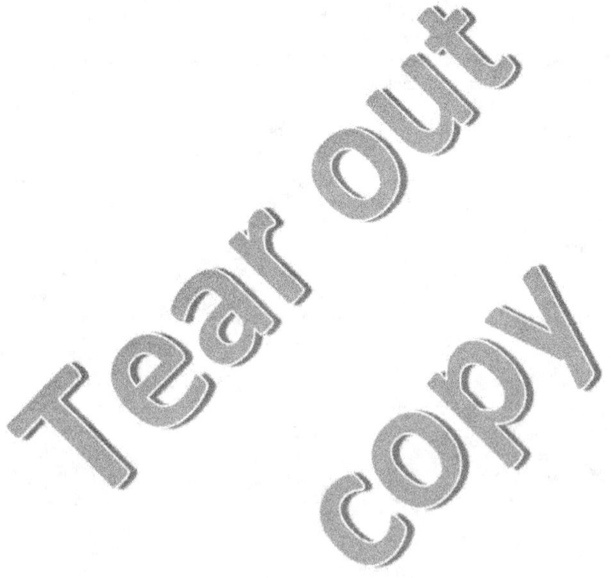

Vegetarian "Like" Example

Meal	Foods	Est. Calories
Day 1		**1103**
Morning	2 Eggs, Hard Boiled	144
Lunch	Beans, baked (1 cup)	239
Lunch	Corn on the cob	155
Lunch	Papayas (1 cup)	62
Snack	Sunflower seeds (1 oz)	140
Dinner	Firm Tofu (6 oz)	195
Dinner	Peppers, sweet, green (1 cup)	30
Dinner	Cabbage (1 cup)	19
Dinner	Red Potato, baked (small 1" dia)	57
Snack	Papayas (1 cup)	62
Day 2		**1082**
Morning	1 Egg, fried in olive oil	90
Snack	Carrots, baby (8)	35
Lunch	Beans, baked (1 cup)	239
Lunch	Peppers, sweet, red (1 cup)	46
Lunch	2 Plums	76
Snack	Nuts, almonds (~14)	85
Dinner	Sunflower seeds (1 oz)	140
Dinner	Vegetarian soup	178
Dinner	Tomatoes (1 cup)	25
Dinner	Yogurt (6oz)	106
Snack	No butter popcorn, 2 cups	62
Day 3		**1138**
Morning	Mangos, raw	99
Morning	Raspberries, raw 1 cup	64
Snack	Nuts, almonds (~14)	85
Lunch	Firm Tofu (6 oz)	195
Lunch	Corn on the cob	155
Lunch	Cabbage (2 cup)	39
Lunch	Spinach, cooked (1 cup)	41
Snack	Papayas (1 cup)	62
Dinner	Cabbage (1 cup)	19
Dinner	Vegetarian Burgers	246
Dinner	Peppers, sweet, green (1 cup)	30
Dinner	Red Potato, baked (small 1" dia)	57
Snack	Peppers, sweet, red (1 cup)	46

Meal	Food	Est. Calories
Day 4		**1131**
Morning	Blackberries, raw 1 cup	62
Morning	1 Egg, fried in olive oil	90
Snack	Nuts, almonds (~14)	85
Lunch	Vegetarian soup	178
Lunch	Yogurt (6oz)	106
Lunch	Cabbage (2 cup)	39
Lunch	Corn on the cob	155
Snack	Carrots, baby (8)	35
Dinner	Beans, baked (1 cup)	239
Dinner	Spinach, cooked (1 cup)	41
Dinner	Tomatoes (1 cup)	25
Snack	2 Plums	76
Day 5 & 7		**1109**
Morning	2 Eggs, Hard Boiled	144
Morning	Mangos, raw	99
Snack	Nuts, almonds (~14)	85
Snack	Raspberries, raw 1 cup	64
Lunch	Beans, baked (1 cup)	239
Lunch	Papayas (1 cup)	62
Snack	Raspberries, raw 1 cup	64
Dinner	Firm Tofu (6 oz)	195
Dinner	Peppers, sweet, green (1 cup)	30
Dinner	Red Potato, baked (small 1" dia)	57
Snack	Carrots, baby (16)	70
Day 6		**1136**
Morning	1 Egg, fried in olive oil	90
Snack	Plums, raw	76
Lunch	Corn on the cob	155
Lunch	Vegetarian Burgers	246
Lunch	Carrots, baby (8)	35
Lunch	Spinach, cooked (1 cup)	41
Snack	Nuts, almonds (~14)	85
Dinner	Vegetarian soup	178
Dinner	Peppers, sweet, red (1 cup)	46
Dinner	Cabbage (1 cup)	19
Dinner	Tomatoes (1 cup)	25
Snack	Sunflower seeds (1 oz)	140

Shopping List

Item	Qty	Item	Qty	Item	Qty
Eggs	9 large	Yogurt, Greek, non fat	12 oz	Bell Peppers, green	4 cups
Mangos	3	Sunflower seeds	3 oz	Cabbage, raw	7 cups
Papayas	5	Nuts, almonds	3 oz	Spinach, Frozen	3 cups
Plums	4	Soup, vegetarian canned	6 cups	Tomatoes	3 cups
Blackberries	1 cups	Red Potato, baked (small 1	4		
Raspberries	5 cups	No butter popcorn	1 Bags		
Vegetarian Burger	2	Peppers, sweet, red	2 pepper		
Beans, baked	5 cup	Carrots, baby	1 Bags		
Firm Tofu	24 oz	Corn on the cob	4 cob		

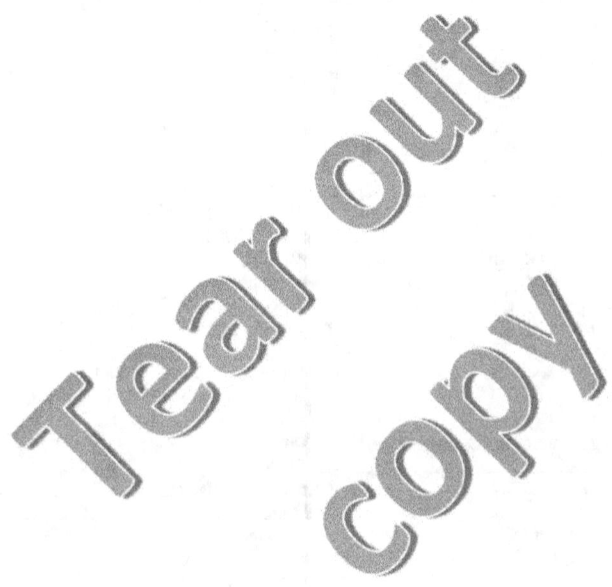
Tear out copy

Paleo Diet Example

Meal	Foods	Est. Calories
Day 1		1158
Morning	Peaches (med.)	60
Morning	Egg, whole, cooked, fried in olive oil	90
Snack	Grapes, red or green (1 cup)	104
Lunch	Beef, grass-fed, loin steak (3 oz)	169
Lunch	Asparagus (1 cup)	32
Lunch	Spinach, cooked, boiled (1 cup)	41
Lunch	Apple (med.) & Cabbage (1 cup)	84
Snack	Nuts, cashew nuts (1 oz)	157
Dinner	Chicken breast, skinless, grilled (3oz)	128
Dinner	Peppers, sweet, green (1 cup)	30
Dinner	Squash, butternut, cooked (1 cup)	82
Dinner	Blueberries (1cup) & Papayas (1cup)	146
Snack	Carrots, baby (8)	35
Day 2		1180
Morning	Orange (med.)	81
Morning	Egg, whole, cooked, Hard Boiled	72
Snack	Sunflower seeds (1 oz)	140
Lunch	Fish, salmon (3 oz)	121
Lunch	Broccoli (2 cups) & Strawberries (1c)	111
Lunch	Sweet potato, baked (med)	105
Snack	Carrots, baby (8)	35
Dinner	Pork, loin, trimmed (3 oz)	134
Dinner	Carrots, baby (16)	70
Dinner	1/2 Banana	100
Dinner	Cauliflower (2 cups)	54
Snack	Nuts, cashew nuts (1 oz)	157
Day 3		1158
Morning	Orange (med.)	84
Morning	Egg, whole, cooked, fried in olive oil	90
Snack	Carrots, baby (8)	35
Lunch	Chicken breast, skinless, grilled (3oz)	128
Lunch	Asparagus (1 cup)	32
Lunch	Spinach, cooked, boiled (1 cup)	41
Lunch	Apple (med.) & Papayas (1 cup)	127
Snack	Grapes, red or green (1 cup)	104
Dinner	Beef, grass-fed, loin steak (3 oz)	169
Dinner	Peppers, sweet, green (1 cup)	30
Dinner	Cabbage (1 cup) & Peaches (med.)	79
Dinner	Squash, butternut, cooked (1 cup)	82
Snack	Nuts, cashew nuts (1 oz)	157

Meal	Food	Est. Calories
Day 4		1192
Morning	Apple (med.)	65
Morning	Egg, whole, cooked, Hard Boiled	72
Snack	Sunflower seeds (1 oz)	140
Lunch	Pork, loin, trimmed (3 oz)	134
Lunch	Broccoli (2 cups)	62
Lunch	1/2 Banana	100
Lunch	Sweet potato, baked (med)	105
Snack	Carrots, baby (8)	35
Dinner	Fish, salmon (3 oz)	121
Dinner	Carrots, baby 16 & Strawberries (1c)	119
Dinner	Cauliflower (2 cups)	54
Dinner	Orange (med.)	81
Snack	Grapes, red or green (1 cup)	104
Day 5 & 7		1194
Morning	Orange (med.)	81
Morning	Egg, whole, cooked, fried in olive oil	90
Snack	Carrots, baby (8)	35
Lunch	Beef, grass-fed, loin steak (3 oz)	169
Lunch	1/2 Banana & Asparagus (1 cup)	132
Lunch	Spinach, cooked, boiled (1 cup)	41
Lunch	Apple (med.)	65
Snack	Grapes, red or green (1 cup)	104
Dinner	Pork, loin, trimmed (3 oz)	134
Dinner	Carrots, baby (16) & Cauliflower 2c	124
Dinner	Cabbage (1 cup) & Peaches (med.)	79
Snack	Sunflower seeds (1 oz)	140
Day 6		1189
Morning	Orange (med.)	81
Morning	Egg, whole, cooked, Hard Boiled	72
Snack	Carrots, baby (8)	35
Lunch	Fish, salmon (3 oz)	121
Lunch	Broccoli (2 cups) & Papayas (1 cup)	124
Lunch	Sweet potato, baked (med)	105
Snack	Nuts, cashew nuts (1 oz)	157
Dinner	Chicken breast, skinless, grilled (3oz)	128
Dinner	Peppers, sweet, green (1 cup)	30
Dinner	Strawberries (1 cup)	49
Dinner	Squash, butternut, cooked (1 cup)	82
Dinner	Apple (med.)	65
Snack	Sunflower seeds (1 oz)	140

Shopping List

Egg	7 large	Pork, loin,	12 oz	Asparagus	4 cups
Apples	6	Beef, grass-fed, loin steak	12 oz	Bell Peppers, green, raw	3 cups
Bananas	2	Fish, salmon	9 oz	Broccoli	6 cups
Oranges	6	Chicken, breast, skinless	9 oz	Cabbage, savoy, raw	4 cups
Papayas	3	Nuts, cashew nuts, raw	4 oz	Cauliflower	8 cups
Peaches	4	Sunflower seeds	5 oz	Spinach, Frozen	4 cups
Blueberries	1 cups	Squash, butternut	3 cups		
Grapes	5 cups	Sweet potato, baked (med	3		
Strawberries	3 cups	Carrots, baby	3 Bags		

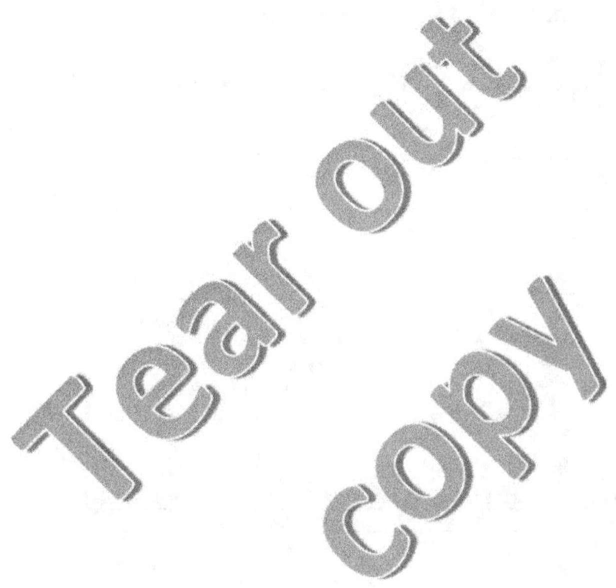

Tear out copy

Higher Protein Week Example

Meal	Foods	Est. Calories	Meal	Food	Est. Calories
Day 1		1523	**Day 4**		1420
Morning	Ham, 3 slices (2 oz)	69	Morning	Turkey, 3 slices,	81
Morning	2 Eggs, cooked, Hard Boiled	144	Morning	2 Eggs, cooked, fried in olive oil	180
Snack	Yogurt, Greek, (6oz)	100	Snack	Carrots, baby (16)	70
Lunch	Beef, steaks, chopped (6oz)	526	Lunch	Beef, tenderloin 6oz &Broccoli 2cups	336
Lunch	Cheese, cream, (1 tbsp)	19	Lunch	Peppers, sweet, red (1 cup)	46
Lunch	Turkey, 3 slices,	81	Lunch	Spinach, cooked, boiled (1 cup)	41
Snack	Shrimp, cooked (6oz)	168	Lunch	Bacon, cooked (2 slices)	108
Dinner	Bacon, cooked (2 slices)	108	Snack	Yogurt, Greek, (6oz)	106
Dinner	Pork, loin, trimmed (4 oz)	195	Dinner	Peppers, sweet, yellow (1 cup)	50
Dinner	Sour cream, (1 tbsp)	9	Dinner	Fish, salmon (4 oz)	161
Snack	Cheese, cottage, (1 cup)	104	Dinner	Asparagus (2 cups) & Shrimp (3oz)	148
Day 2		1541	Dinner	Squash, zucchini (1 cup)	66
Morning	Bacon, cooked (2 slices)	108	Snack	Cauliflower, raw (1 cup)	27
Morning	2 Eggs, cooked, fried in olive oil	180	**Day 5 & 7**		1499
snack	1cup red pepper &Asparagus 2cups	110	Morning	Bacon, cooked (2 slices)	108
Lunch	Fish, salmon (4 oz)	161	Morning	2 Eggs, cooked, Hard Boiled	144
Lunch	Broccoli (2 cups) & Shrimp (6oz)	146	Snack	Yogurt, Greek, (6oz)	106
Lunch	Shrimp, cooked (3oz)	84	Lunch	Beef, steaks, chopped (6oz)	526
Lunch	Spinach, cooked, boiled (1 cup)	41	Snack	Shrimp, cooked (6oz)	168
Snack	Yogurt, Greek, non fat (6oz)	106	Dinner	Beef, tenderloin (6 oz)	274
Dinner	Beef, tenderloin (6 oz)	274	Dinner	Ham, 3 slices (2 oz)	69
Dinner	Shrimp, cooked (6oz)	168	Snack	Cheese, cottage, (1 cup)	104
Dinner	Squash, zucchini (1 cup)	66	**Day 6**		1482
Dinner	Turkey, 3 slices,	81	Morning	Bacon, cooked (2 slices)	108
Snack	Celery (3-5" sticks)	16	Morning	2 Eggs, cooked, fried in olive oil	180
Day 3		1529	Snack	Cheese, cottage, (1 cup)	104
Morning	Bacon, cooked (2 slices)	108	Snack	Carrots, baby (16)	70
Morning	2 Eggs, cooked, Hard Boiled	144	Lunch	Broccoli (2 cups) & Salmon 4oz	223
Snack	Yogurt, Greek, (6oz)	106	Lunch	Spinach, cooked, boiled (1 cup)	41
Lunch	Pork, loin, trimmed (4 oz)	195	Lunch	Turkey, 3 slices,	81
Lunch	Cheese, cottage, (1 cup)	104	Snack	Yogurt, Greek, (6oz)	106
Lunch	Turkey, 3 slices,	81	Dinner	Pork, loin, trimmed (4 oz)	195
Snack	Shrimp, cooked (6oz)	168	Dinner	Cauliflower (2 cups) & Shrimp (6oz)	222
Dinner	Beef, steaks, chopped (6oz)	526	Dinner	Sour cream, (1 tbsp)	9
Dinner	Sour cream, (1 tbsp)	9	Dinner	Bacon, cooked (2 slices)	108
Dinner	Ham, 3 slices (2 oz)	69	Snack	Celery (3-5" sticks) & cream cheese	35
Snack	Cheese, cream, 1 tbsp	19			

Shopping List

Bacon (sugar free)	16 slices	Cheese, cream,	3 tbsp	Spinach, Frozen	3 cups
Eggs	14 large	Sour cream,	3 tablesp	Squash, zucchini	2 cups
Ham, sliced,	10 oz	Shrimp, cooked	42 oz	Peppers, sweet, red	2 pepper
Turkey, sliced,	15 slices	Yogurt, Greek,	42 oz	Peppers, sweet,yellow	1 pepper
Beef, tenderloin	4 fillets	Celery, raw	2 Stocks		
Beef, steak	24 oz	Carrots, baby	1 Bags		
Fish, salmon	12 oz	Asparagus	4 cups		
Pork, loin,	12 oz	Broccoli	6 cups		
Cheese, cottage,	5 cup	Cauliflower, raw	3 cups		

Low-Calorie Week Example

Day 1:	885 total calories	~Cal.	Day 2:	885 total calories	~Cal.
Breakfast	Orange & Coffee/Tea	70	Breakfast	Apple, Coffee/Tea	70
Snack	Melba Toast (15 grams) ~3 pcs	60	Snacks	Orange	70
Lunch	Grilled Chicken (4 oz)	130	Lunch	Hamburger (3 oz) 93% lean, no bun	150
Lunch Side	Spinach (6oz) & Yogurt	140	Lunch Side	Cauliflower (6oz) & Light Soup	140
Lunch Side	Strawberries (6 oz. or 6-7)	45	Lunch Side	Strawberries (6 oz)	45
Dinner	Tilapia (3.5oz)	100	Dinner	Shrimp (3.5oz)	110
Dinner Sides	Broccoli (6oz) & Baked Potato	170	Dinner Side	Asparagus (7oz) & Baked Potato	130
Snack	Apple (medium) & Light Soup	170	Snack	Tomatoes (7oz) & Yogurt	140

Day 3 & 5:	875 total calories	~Cal.	Day 4:	845 total calories	~Cal.
Breakfast	Orange, Coffee/Tea	70	Breakfast	Strawberries, Coffee/Tea	45
Snacks	Melba Toast (10 grams) & yogurt	140	Snacks	Yogurt	100
Lunch	Chicken (4 oz)	130	Lunch	Sirloin Steak (3oz) & Potato	260
Lunch Side	Broccoli (6oz) & Potato	160	Lunch Side	Spinach Salad (no calorie dressing)	40
Lunch Side	Salad (no calorie dressing) & Apple	100	Lunch Side	Orange & Light soup	170
Dinner	Tilapia (3.5oz)	100	Dinner	Chicken (4 oz)	130
Dinner Sides	Cauliflower(6oz) & Light Soup	140	Dinner Side	Celery (7oz)	30
Snack	Strawberries (6-7)	45	Snack	Apple (medium)	70

Day 6:	895 total calories	~Cal.	Day 7	875 total calories	~Cal.
Breakfast	Strawberries (6-7), Coffee/Tea	45	Breakfast	Coffee/Tea & Apple	70
Snacks	Orange	70	Snacks	Melba Toast (10 grams)	40
Lunch	Sirloin Steak (3oz)	160	Lunch	Hamburger (3 oz) 93% lean, no bun	150
Lunch Side	Cauliflower(6oz)	40	Lunch Side	Celery (7oz) & Light soup	130
Lunch Side	Tomatoes (7oz) & Yogurt	140	Lunch Side	Strawberries 6 oz. or 6-7	45
Dinner	Tilapia (3.5oz) & Potato	200	Dinner	Shrimp (3.5oz)	110
Dinner Sides	Asparagus (7oz) & Melba Toast (10 g)	80	Dinner Side	Broccoli (6oz) & Potato	160
Snack	Apple & Light Soup	170	Snack	Orange & Yogurt	170

Fruits & Veggies		*Veggies*		*Meats*		*Snacks*	
• Oranges	7	• Celery	1 bunch	• Tilapia	14 oz	• Melba Toast	1box
• Apples	7	• Asparagus	14oz	• Chicken	16oz	• Tea packets	1box
• Strawberries	3 lbs	• Broccoli	2-12oz bags	• Sirloin Steak	6oz	• Coffee	1bag
• Tomatoes	2lb	• Cauliflower	2-12oz bags	• Lean Beef	6oz	• Yogurt	7
• Lettuce	1 bag	• Spinach	1 bag	• Shrimp	7oz	• Light Soup	4cans
		• Small Potatoes	1 bag				

**Light Soup would be one that is ~100 calories or less per serving.

Simple Week Example

Meal	Foods	Est. Calories	Meal	Food	Est. Calories
Day 1		1196	**Day 4**		1183
Snack	Snacks, beef jerky, (1oz)	116	Morning	Blackberries, raw 1 cup	62
Morning	1 Hard Boiled Egg	72	Morning	2 Eggs, Hard Boiled	144
Snack	Snacks, popcorn, microwave, low fat	120	Snack	Nuts, almonds (~14)	85
Lunch	Chicken breast, mesquite (3oz)	102	Lunch	Cauliflower (2 cups) & Turkey, 3 slice	135
Lunch	Asparagus (1 cup)	32	Lunch	Lettuce, 2 cups	20
Lunch	Nonfat cottage cheese 1cup	104	Lunch	Dressing, fat-free	51
Lunch	French fries (3 oz)	117	Lunch	Raspberries, raw & Spinach, cooked (	105
Lunch	Blackberries, raw 1 cup	62	Snack	Carrots, baby (8)	35
Dinner	Fish, tilapia (3 oz) & Shrimp, cooked (	195	Snack	Snacks, beef jerky, (1oz)	116
Dinner	Lettuce, 2 cups	20	Dinner	Pork, loin, trimmed (3 oz)	134
Dinner	Dressing, fat-free	51	Dinner	Broccoli (2 cups)	62
Dinner	Raspberries, raw 1 cup	64	Dinner	White potato, baked (med)	114
Snack	Carrots, baby (8) & Yogurt (6oz)	141	Snack	Snacks, popcorn, microwave, low fat	120
Day 2		1197	**Day 5 & 7**		1118
Morning	2 Eggs, fried in olive oil	182	Morning	1 Hard Boiled Egg & Raspberries, raw	88
Snack	Nuts, almonds (~14)	85	Snack	Carrots, baby (8)	35
Lunch	Pork, loin, trimmed (4 oz)	195	Snack	Snacks, beef jerky, (1oz)	116
Lunch	Cauliflower (2 cups)	54	Lunch	Chicken breast, mesquite (3oz)	102
Lunch	Dressing, fat-free	51	Lunch	Asparagus (1 cup)	32
Dinner	Lettuce, 2 cups	20	Lunch	French fries (3 oz)	117
Lunch	Spinach, cooked (1 cup)	41	Lunch	Blackberries, raw 1 cup	62
Snack	Carrots, baby (8)	35	Snack	Snacks, popcorn, microwave, low fat	120
Dinner	Turkey, 6 slices (4 oz)	190	Dinner	Broccoli (2 cups) & Turkey, 3 slices	143
Dinner	Broccoli (2 cups)	62	Dinner	Nonfat cottage cheese 1cup	104
Dinner	White potato, baked (med)	114	Dinner	White potato, baked (med)	114
Dinner	Blackberries, raw 1 cup	62	Snack	Nuts, almonds (~14)	85
Snack	Yogurt (6oz)	106	**Day 6**		1111
Day 3		1129	Morning	2 Eggs, Hard Boiled	144
Morning	Raspberries, raw 1 cup	64	Snack	Carrots, baby (8)	35
Snack	Avocados, raw (.5 cup) & Yogurt (6oz	226	Lunch	Pork, loin, trimmed (3 oz)	134
Morning	1 Hard Boiled Egg	72	Lunch	Cauliflower (2 cups)	54
Snack	Carrots, baby (8)	35	Lunch	Shrimp, cooked (3oz)	84
Lunch	Fish, tilapia (3 oz)	111	Lunch	Blackberries, raw & Spinach, cooked	103
Lunch	Asparagus (1 cup) & Shrimp, cooked	116	Snack	Avocados, raw (.5 cup) & Yogurt (6oz	226
Lunch	French fries (3 oz)	117	Dinner	Fish, tilapia (3 oz)	111
Lunch	Blackberries, raw 1 cup	62	Dinner	Lettuce, 2 cups	20
Dinner	Chicken breast, mesquite (3oz)	102	Dinner	Dressing, fat-free	51
Dinner	Nonfat cottage cheese 1cup	104	Dinner	Raspberries, raw 1 cup	64
Snack	Snacks, popcorn, microwave, low fat	120	Snack	Nuts, almonds (~14)	85

Shopping List

Eggs	10 large	Dressing, fat-free	8 tbsp	Avocados	1		
Blackberries	7 cups	Shrimp, cooked	9 oz	Carrots, baby	2 Bags		
Raspberries	6 cups	Yogurt, Greek, non fat	24 oz	Asparagus	4 cups		
Turkey, low-fat, Sliced	6 oz	Nuts, almonds (~14)	3 oz	Broccoli	8 cups		
Fish, tilapia	3 fillet	Snacks, beef jerky	4 oz	Cauliflower, raw	6 cups		
Chicken Breast, mesquite,	12 ounce	Snacks, popcorn, microwav	5 oz	Lettuce	8 cups		
Pork, loin,	10 oz	White potato, baked (med)	4 med.				
Turkey, low-fat, Sliced	4 oz	Frozen french fries	12 oz				
Cheese, cottage, nonfat	4 cup	Spinach, Frozen	3 cups				

Vegetarian "Like" Example

Meal	Foods	Est. Calories
Day 1		**1103**
Morning	2 Eggs, Hard Boiled	144
Lunch	Beans, baked (1 cup)	239
Lunch	Corn on the cob	155
Lunch	Papayas (1 cup)	62
Snack	Sunflower seeds (1 oz)	140
Dinner	Firm Tofu (6 oz)	195
Dinner	Peppers, sweet, green (1 cup)	30
Dinner	Cabbage (1 cup)	19
Dinner	Red Potato, baked (small 1" dia)	57
Snack	Papayas (1 cup)	62
Day 2		**1082**
Morning	1 Egg, fried in olive oil	90
Snack	Carrots, baby (8)	35
Lunch	Beans, baked (1 cup)	239
Lunch	Peppers, sweet, red (1 cup)	46
Lunch	2 Plums	76
Snack	Nuts, almonds (~14)	85
Dinner	Sunflower seeds (1 oz)	140
Dinner	Vegetarian soup	178
Dinner	Tomatoes (1 cup)	25
Dinner	Yogurt (6oz)	106
Snack	No butter popcorn, 2 cups	62
Day 3		**1138**
Morning	Mangos, raw	99
Morning	Raspberries, raw 1 cup	64
Snack	Nuts, almonds (~14)	85
Lunch	Firm Tofu (6 oz)	195
Lunch	Corn on the cob	155
Lunch	Cabbage (2 cup)	39
Lunch	Spinach, cooked (1 cup)	41
Snack	Papayas (1 cup)	62
Dinner	Cabbage (1 cup)	19
Dinner	Vegetarian Burgers	246
Dinner	Peppers, sweet, green (1 cup)	30
Dinner	Red Potato, baked (small 1" dia)	57
Snack	Peppers, sweet, red (1 cup)	46

Meal	Food	Est. Calories
Day 4		**1131**
Morning	Blackberries, raw 1 cup	62
Morning	1 Egg, fried in olive oil	90
Snack	Nuts, almonds (~14)	85
Lunch	Vegetarian soup	178
Lunch	Yogurt (6oz)	106
Lunch	Cabbage (2 cup)	39
Lunch	Corn on the cob	155
Snack	Carrots, baby (8)	35
Dinner	Beans, baked (1 cup)	239
Dinner	Spinach, cooked (1 cup)	41
Dinner	Tomatoes (1 cup)	25
Snack	2 Plums	76
Day 5 & 7		**1109**
Morning	2 Eggs, Hard Boiled	144
Morning	Mangos, raw	99
Snack	Nuts, almonds (~14)	85
Snack	Raspberries, raw 1 cup	64
Lunch	Beans, baked (1 cup)	239
Lunch	Papayas (1 cup)	62
Snack	Raspberries, raw 1 cup	64
Dinner	Firm Tofu (6 oz)	195
Dinner	Peppers, sweet, green (1 cup)	30
Dinner	Red Potato, baked (small 1" dia)	57
Snack	Carrots, baby (16)	70
Day 6		**1136**
Morning	1 Egg, fried in olive oil	90
Snack	Plums, raw	76
Lunch	Corn on the cob	155
Lunch	Vegetarian Burgers	246
Lunch	Carrots, baby (8)	35
Lunch	Spinach, cooked (1 cup)	41
Snack	Nuts, almonds (~14)	85
Dinner	Vegetarian soup	178
Dinner	Peppers, sweet, red (1 cup)	46
Dinner	Cabbage (1 cup)	19
Dinner	Tomatoes (1 cup)	25
Snack	Sunflower seeds (1 oz)	140

Shopping List

Eggs	9 large	Yogurt, Greek, non fat	12 oz	Bell Peppers, green	4 cups
Mangos	3	Sunflower seeds	3 oz	Cabbage, raw	7 cups
Papayas	5	Nuts, almonds	3 oz	Spinach, Frozen	3 cups
Plums	4	Soup, vegetarian canned	6 cups	Tomatoes	3 cups
Blackberries	1 cups	Red Potato, baked (small	4		
Raspberries	5 cups	No butter popcorn	1 Bags		
Vegetarian Burger	2	Peppers, sweet, red	2 pepper		
Beans, baked	5 cup	Carrots, baby	1 Bags		
Firm Tofu	24 oz	Corn on the cob	4 cob		

Paleo Diet Example

Meal	Foods	Est. Calories	Meal	Food	Est. Calories
Day 1		1158	**Day 4**		1192
Morning	Peaches (med.)	60	**Morning**	Apple (med.)	65
Morning	Egg, whole, cooked, fried in olive oil	90	**Morning**	Egg, whole, cooked, Hard Boiled	72
Snack	Grapes, red or green (1 cup)	104	Snack	Sunflower seeds (1 oz)	140
Lunch	Beef, grass-fed, loin steak (3 oz)	169	**Lunch**	Pork, loin, trimmed (3 oz)	134
Lunch	Asparagus (1 cup)	32	**Lunch**	Broccoli (2 cups)	62
Lunch	Spinach, cooked, boiled (1 cup)	41	**Lunch**	1/2 Banana	100
Lunch	Apple (med.) & Cabbage (1 cup)	84	**Lunch**	Sweet potato, baked (med)	105
Snack	Nuts, cashew nuts (1 oz)	157	Snack	Carrots, baby (8)	35
Dinner	Chicken breast, skinless, grilled (3oz)	128	**Dinner**	Fish, salmon (3 oz)	121
Dinner	Peppers, sweet, green (1 cup)	30	**Dinner**	Carrots, baby 16 & Strawberries (1c)	119
Dinner	Squash, butternut, cooked (1 cup)	82	**Dinner**	Cauliflower (2 cups)	54
Dinner	Blueberries (1cup) & Papayas (1cup)	146	**Dinner**	Orange (med.)	81
Snack	Carrots, baby (8)	35	Snack	Grapes, red or green (1 cup)	104
Day 2		1180	**Day 5 & 7**		1194
Morning	Orange (med.)	81	**Morning**	Orange (med.)	81
Morning	Egg, whole, cooked, Hard Boiled	72	**Morning**	Egg, whole, cooked, fried in olive oil	90
Snack	Sunflower seeds (1 oz)	140	Snack	Carrots, baby (8)	35
Lunch	Fish, salmon (3 oz)	121	**Lunch**	Beef, grass-fed, loin steak (3 oz)	169
Lunch	Broccoli (2 cups) & Strawberries (1c)	111	**Lunch**	1/2 Banana & Asparagus (1 cup)	132
Lunch	Sweet potato, baked (med)	105	**Lunch**	Spinach, cooked, boiled (1 cup)	41
Snack	Carrots, baby (8)	35	**Lunch**	Apple (med.)	65
Dinner	Pork, loin, trimmed (3 oz)	134	Snack	Grapes, red or green (1 cup)	104
Dinner	Carrots, baby (16)	70	**Dinner**	Pork, loin, trimmed (3 oz)	134
Dinner	1/2 Banana	100	**Dinner**	Carrots, baby (16) & Cauliflower 2c	124
Dinner	Cauliflower (2 cups)	54	**Dinner**	Cabbage (1 cup) & Peaches (med.)	79
Snack	Nuts, cashew nuts (1 oz)	157	Snack	Sunflower seeds (1 oz)	140
Day 3		1158	**Day 6**		1189
Morning	Orange (med.)	84	**Morning**	Orange (med.)	81
Morning	Egg, whole, cooked, fried in olive oil	90	**Morning**	Egg, whole, cooked, Hard Boiled	72
Snack	Carrots, baby (8)	35	Snack	Carrots, baby (8)	35
Lunch	Chicken breast, skinless, grilled (3oz)	128	**Lunch**	Fish, salmon (3 oz)	121
Lunch	Asparagus (1 cup)	32	**Lunch**	Broccoli (2 cups) & Papayas (1 cup)	124
Lunch	Spinach, cooked, boiled (1 cup)	41	**Lunch**	Sweet potato, baked (med)	105
Lunch	Apple (med.) & Papayas (1 cup)	127	Snack	Nuts, cashew nuts (1 oz)	157
Snack	Grapes, red or green (1 cup)	104	**Dinner**	Chicken breast, skinless, grilled (3oz)	128
Dinner	Beef, grass-fed, loin steak (3 oz)	169	**Dinner**	Peppers, sweet, green (1 cup)	30
Dinner	Peppers, sweet, green (1 cup)	30	**Dinner**	Strawberries (1 cup)	49
Dinner	Cabbage (1 cup) & Peaches (med.)	79	**Dinner**	Squash, butternut, cooked (1 cup)	82
Dinner	Squash, butternut, cooked (1 cup)	82	**Dinner**	Apple (med.)	65
Snack	Nuts, cashew nuts (1 oz)	157	Snack	Sunflower seeds (1 oz)	140

Shopping List

Egg	7 large	Pork, loin,	12 oz	Asparagus	4 cups
Apples	6	Beef, grass-fed, loin steak	12 oz	Bell Peppers, green, raw	3 cups
Bananas	2	Fish, salmon	9 oz	Broccoli	6 cups
Oranges	6	Chicken, breast, skinless	9 oz	Cabbage, savoy, raw	4 cups
Papayas	3	Nuts, cashew nuts, raw	4 oz	Cauliflower	8 cups
Peaches	4	Sunflower seeds	5 oz	Spinach, Frozen	4 cups
Blueberries	1 cups	Squash, butternut	3 cups		
Grapes	5 cups	Sweet potato, baked (med	3		
Strawberries	3 cups	Carrots, baby	3 Bags		

CHAPTER 11: NEXT STEPS

What now?

At the end this challenge you have several different menu plans so that you have enough for the next few weeks. You also have access to our Preferred Members Area, by just emailing me at pam@3weekslimdownchallenge.com, where we provide you with even more menus, books, and tools to support you.

Want to do the challenge again?

Check with me and I'll send you a promo code for a discount on another book.

You can start your "do-over" next week, next month, or tomorrow. Your choice.

You are awesome!!! Just because this challenge is over, doesn't mean I'm done supporting you to be the best you can be. Post on our Facebook Group whenever you need motivation, and I will ensure you get it.

<u>Last Challenge</u>

- Share your results and encourage others on their journey. Brag about your success, you deserve it.

ABOUT THE AUTHOR

I'm a busy working mom of 3 amazing kids, focused on staying at a "healthy" weight. My main goal is to simplify what is working so that you can save time and money while getting healthy. Losing weight is hard enough without making it more complicated than it needs to be. I don't have time to mess around with all the fad diets. I just want real, simple, fast, and healthy foods.

If you follow my blog, you'll know my goal is not to be "thin", but to be healthy. I love to go to Colorado and hike. In fact, I was up at the top of Herman's Peak a few years back. A 14,000-foot mountain is a great way to bond with your children. It feels so good to be healthy enough to do those things with my kids. My personal health inspired these menu plans, but my readers stories inspire me every day to continue to create more to serve you.

3weekslimdownchallenge.com